101 HACKS OF STAYING YOUNG
AND LONG LIFE SECRETS

HOW NOT TO FADE OUT

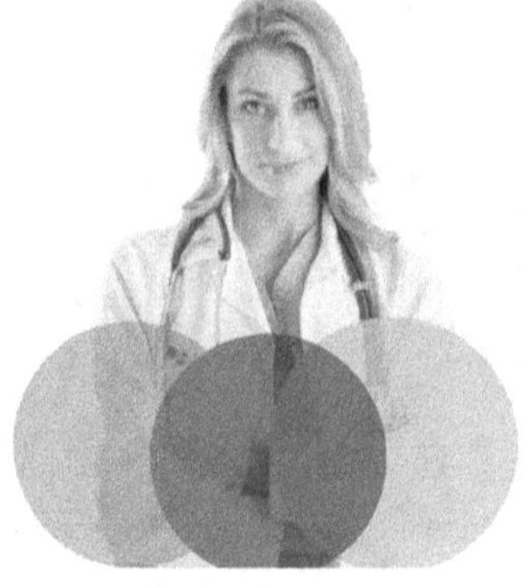

About the Author

In a world where time is our most precious commodity, "How not to fade out"- 101 Hacks of staying young and long life secrets" is your guide to mastering the art of longevity. With a zest for life that's infectious, I have traveled the globe, delving into diverse cultures, and uncovering the secrets to living a life not only long but vibrantly young and healthy. My approach to long life and staying young is about embracing the beauty of existence, savoring every moment, and nurturing your health along the way.

By the way, I am **Dr. Micheal Edward (MD),** passionate advocate for health and well-being, dedicated to helping individuals live longer, younger healthier lives. I have spent years researching and educating people about the principles of longevity, balanced living, and the science of a healthy, fulfilling life. I understand that the journey to a longer and healthier life is not a one-size-fits-all endeavor and so, I have tailored this book to offer a wealth of practical advice, backed by the latest research, to guide you on your path.

In a quest for secrets for long life, health and wellness, I have had several journeys from the bustling streets of the United States, Tokyo to the serene villages of the Mediterranean, and the wisdom gathered along the way is at the heart of this ebook.

In an attempt to crack the code to longevity, I will be sharing the keys to longevity, secrets that can't be found in a lab or a textbook with you shortly. The pages you're about to explore are a tapestry woven with the threads of ancient wisdom, modern science, and my unique experiences.

On a lighter note, whenever I am not researching, writing, or on a new adventure, you can easily find me in the kitchen, creating delectable dishes that are as much a feast for the senses as they are for the body. I believe that food should be a celebration of life, and every meal is a chance to nurture your body and soul.

As you delve into the pages of this book, you're not just getting advice from a health expert; you're embarking on a journey with a trusted friend and guide. Let's explore the world of longevity together.

Acknowledgments

Of a truth, my journey to unlocking the secrets of longevity and well-being would not have been possible without the support, wisdom, and inspiration of many individuals and communities. I want to express my heartfelt gratitude to those who have contributed to this work in various ways.

To My Family and Wife, Emily Edward:

Thank you for your unwavering support, love, and encouragement. You have been the foundation of my life's journey and the source of my strength and inspiration.

To My Friends:

I'm honestly grateful to friends, camaraderie who shared experiences that have added rich textures to this book and have often been a source of motivation and laughter.

To My Mentors:

I'm indebted to those who have shared their knowledge and guided me on this path. Your wisdom and expertise have been invaluable.

To the Researchers and Experts:

I'm grateful for the scientists, medical professionals, and experts who have dedicated their careers to advancing our understanding of health and well-being. Your research has paved the way for this book.

To the Communities I've Encountered:

From the vibrant Blue Zones to the serene meditation retreats, the cultures and communities I've encountered during my explorations have taught me invaluable lessons about life, health, and happiness.

To the Readers:

You, the readers, are the ultimate reason for this book's existence. Thank you for joining me on this journey and for your commitment to a longer, healthier life. It's my hope that this book serves as a guide to a more vibrant, fulfilled existence.

Let's continue to explore the world of well-being and longevity together.

With profound gratitude,

Dr. Micheal Edward (MD)

101 Hacks of Staying Young and Long Life Secrets

Table of Contents

The question is what is a balanced diet? A balanced diet is the diet that provides the body with all the essential nutrients, vitamins, and minerals it needs to function properly. It typically includes a variety of foods from different food groups in the right proportions. A balanced diet typically consists of the following components:

- Proteins: These are essential for building and repairing tissues in the body. Good sources of protein include lean meats, poultry, fish, eggs, dairy products, legumes, and nuts.

- Carbohydrates: Carbohydrates are the body's primary source of energy. Whole grains, fruits, vegetables, and legumes are healthy sources of carbohydrates.

- Fats: Healthy fats are important for energy, cell growth, and the absorption of certain vitamins. Sources of healthy fats include avocados, nuts, seeds, and olive oil.

- Fruits and Vegetables: These are rich in vitamins, minerals, and antioxidants. They play a crucial role in maintaining overall health.

- Dairy or Dairy Alternatives: These provide calcium for strong bones and teeth. Options include milk, yogurt, and fortified plant-based milk alternatives.

- Fiber: Fiber aids digestion, helps maintain a healthy weight, and can lower the risk of certain chronic diseases. It's found in foods like whole grains, fruits, vegetables, and legumes.

- Hydration: Staying properly hydrated is an important part of a balanced diet. Water is essential for various bodily functions.

- Vitamins and Minerals: These are found in various foods and are necessary for the proper functioning of the body. A balanced diet should provide a wide range of these nutrients.

- Moderation: A balanced diet also involves consuming foods high in sugar, salt, and saturated fats in moderation. Excessive consumption of these can lead to health problems.

- Variety: Eating a variety of foods ensures that you get a broad spectrum of nutrients and reduces the risk of nutritional deficiencies.

The Power of Balanced Diet

A balanced diet offers numerous benefits, the following are some of them:

- Nutrient Adequacy: A balanced diet ensures that you're getting a wide range of essential nutrients, including vitamins, minerals, and macronutrients like carbohydrates, protein, and fats, which are vital for overall health and longevity.

- Weight Management: Maintaining a healthy weight is crucial for long-term health. A balanced diet helps in managing weight, reducing the risk of obesity-related health issues like heart disease and diabetes.

- Energy and Vitality: Proper nutrition provides the energy your body needs to function optimally. This is especially important as you age and need sustained energy for daily activities and maintaining an active lifestyle.

- Heart Health: A diet low in saturated and trans fats, and rich in fruits, vegetables, and whole grains, can reduce the risk of heart diseases by maintaining healthy cholesterol levels and blood pressure.

- Gut Health: A balanced diet with plenty of fiber from fruits and vegetables promotes a healthy gut microbiome, which is linked to improved digestion and a strong immune system.

- Bone Health: Adequate calcium and vitamin D from a balanced diet contribute to strong bones and can help prevent conditions like osteoporosis, which becomes more relevant with age.

- Cognitive Function: Nutrient-rich foods, especially those high in antioxidants and omega-3 fatty acids, support cognitive function and may lower the risk of age-related cognitive decline.

- Longevity and Disease Prevention: A balanced diet can reduce the risk of chronic diseases such as cancer, diabetes, and hypertension, potentially extending your lifespan and enhancing the quality of life in your later years.

- Digestive Health: Proper nutrition promotes regular bowel movements, reducing the risk of constipation and related digestive issues.

- Skin Health: Nutrients like vitamins C and E found in a balanced diet contribute to healthy skin and can slow the aging process.

- Improved Immunity: A diet rich in vitamins, minerals, and antioxidants helps strengthen the immune system, reducing the likelihood of infections and illnesses.

- Reduced Inflammation: Certain foods in a balanced diet, such as anti-inflammatory foods like berries, fatty fish, and leafy greens, can help lower chronic inflammation, which is linked to many age-related diseases.

Incorporating a balanced diet is just one of the many "hacks" for a long and healthy life, nourishing your body with the right foods, you can significantly enhance your chances of living a long, vibrant life.

Superfoods for Longevity

"Superfoods" is a term often used to describe foods that are particularly rich in nutrients and believed to provide various health benefits, including supporting longevity. While there is no specific definition of superfoods, many of these foods are packed with vitamins, minerals, antioxidants, and other bioactive compounds that are associated with improved health. These are some superfoods that are often associated with longevity:

- Berries: Blueberries, strawberries, and other berries are rich in antioxidants and phytochemicals, which may help protect cells from damage and reduce the risk of chronic diseases.

- Leafy Greens: Kale, spinach, and other leafy greens are high in vitamins, minerals, and fiber. They are associated with reduced risk of heart disease and certain cancers.

- Fatty Fish: Salmon, mackerel, and sardines are excellent sources of omega-3 fatty acids, which are known for their anti-inflammatory properties and heart-healthy benefits.

- Nuts and Seeds: Almonds, walnuts, chia seeds, and flaxseeds are packed with healthy fats, fiber, and essential nutrients. They can support heart health and weight management.

- Olive Oil: Extra virgin olive oil is rich in monounsaturated fats and antioxidants, making it a key component of the Mediterranean diet, which is linked to longevity and reduced risk of chronic diseases.

- Turmeric: This spice contains curcumin, a compound with powerful anti-inflammatory and antioxidant properties. It is believed to support brain health and reduce the risk of certain age-related conditions.

- Green Tea: Green tea is high in catechins, which have been associated with improved metabolism, heart health, and reduced risk of cancer.

- Legumes: Foods like lentils, chickpeas, and beans are high in fiber, protein, and various vitamins and minerals. They are linked to lower cholesterol levels and better blood sugar control.

- Yogurt: Probiotic-rich yogurt can support gut health and, in turn, the overall immune system. It's also a source of calcium and protein.

- Tomatoes: Tomatoes contain lycopene, an antioxidant that may reduce the risk of certain cancers and support heart health.

- Avocado: Avocado is a source of healthy monounsaturated fats, fiber, and various vitamins. It's linked to heart health and weight management.

- Garlic: Garlic has antioxidant and anti-inflammatory properties and is associated with reduced risk of heart disease and some cancers.

A well-balanced diet that includes a variety of nutrient-rich foods, along with other healthy lifestyle practices, such as regular exercise and stress management, is key to promoting longevity and overall well-being.

Portion Control and Mindful Eating

Portion control and mindful eating are two practices that can help individuals make healthier food choices and maintain a balanced diet. They involve being aware of what and how much you eat, and they can support weight management and overall well-being.

Portion Control

Portion control is the practice of managing the size of the food servings you consume. It involves paying attention to the quantity of food on your plate and eating an appropriate amount to meet your nutritional needs without overindulging.

Benefits of Portion Control

- Helps prevent overeating and weight gain.
- Supports better digestion by avoiding excessive food intake.
- Reduces the risk of consuming too many calories, which can lead to obesity.
- Promotes awareness of portion sizes in restaurants and when preparing meals at home.

Healthy Tips of Portion Control

- Use smaller plates and bowls to visually control portions.
- Read food labels to understand serving sizes and nutritional content.
- Be mindful of portion sizes when eating out, as restaurant servings can often be larger than necessary.
- Practice mindful eating techniques alongside portion control.

Mindful Eating

Mindful eating is an approach to eating that encourages you to pay full attention to the experience of eating, including the taste, texture, and aroma of the food. It also involves being aware of your body's hunger and fullness cues, as well as the emotional and psychological aspects of eating.

Benefits of Mindful Eating

- Promotes a healthier relationship with food.
- Encourages savoring and enjoying food more fully.
- Helps in recognizing and responding to physical hunger and fullness cues.
- Reduces emotional or stress-related eating.
- Supports weight management and can prevent overeating.

Healthy Tips for Mindful Eating

- Eat without distractions, such as TV or smartphones, to focus on your meal.
- Chew food slowly and savor each bite, paying attention to taste and texture.
- Listen to your body's hunger and fullness signals, eating when hungry and stopping when satisfied.
- Be aware of emotional triggers for eating and seek non-food alternatives for comfort or stress relief.
- Keep a food journal to track eating patterns and emotional connections to food.

Both portion control and mindful eating can be used together to create a healthier relationship with food. By understanding and controlling portion sizes and being present during meals, individuals can make more informed food choices, reduce overeating, and enjoy their meals while maintaining or achieving a healthy weight.

Hydration, or maintaining proper fluid balance in the body, is crucial for overall health and well-being. Staying adequately hydrated offers a wide range of benefits, and in the context of longevity and general health, it is especially important. These are some of the key benefits of hydration:

- Regulation of Body Temperature: Adequate hydration helps regulate body temperature, which is essential for normal bodily functions and overall comfort. It helps your body cool down through sweating in hot weather or during physical activity.

- Cognitive Function: Staying hydrated is essential for optimal cognitive function. Dehydration can lead to difficulties with concentration, memory, and mental clarity.

- Digestive Health: Sufficient water intake supports the digestive system by helping to break down food and move it through the gastrointestinal tract. It can reduce the risk of constipation and other digestive issues.

- Joint Health: Hydration helps maintain joint lubrication and cushioning. Proper fluid balance is essential for joint comfort and flexibility.

- Skin Health: Well-hydrated skin is less prone to dryness and premature aging. It can help maintain skin elasticity and a healthy complexion.

- Energy and Physical Performance: Dehydration can lead to fatigue and reduced physical performance. Staying hydrated is essential for maintaining energy levels and endurance, whether you're exercising or simply going about your daily activities.

- Detoxification: Water plays a role in the body's natural detoxification processes. It helps flush out waste products and toxins through urine and sweat.

- Cardiovascular Health: Proper hydration supports heart health by helping maintain adequate blood volume and circulation. It can also help regulate blood pressure.

- Kidney Function: Adequate water intake is necessary for kidney function. It helps the kidneys filter waste and excess substances from the blood to form urine.

- Weight Management: Drinking water before meals can contribute to a feeling of fullness, potentially reducing calorie intake and supporting weight management.

- Reduced Risk of Urinary Tract Infections: Staying well-hydrated can help prevent urinary tract infections by flushing out bacteria from the urinary system.

- Improved Mood: Dehydration can contribute to mood swings, irritability, and feelings of anxiety. Proper hydration can help stabilize your mood.

- Better Immune Function: Hydration supports the immune system by helping to transport immune cells and antibodies throughout the body.

In the context of longevity, maintaining adequate hydration is crucial because dehydration can lead to health problems and complications, especially as we age. It's recommended to drink water regularly throughout the day and pay attention to your body's signals of thirst. The specific amount of water needed can vary depending on factors like age, activity level, and climate, but generally, drinking around 8 glasses (64 ounces) of water a day is a common guideline.

The Role of Supplements

Supplements play a specific and complementary role in a person's diet and health, particularly when there are deficiencies or specific needs that cannot be met through regular food consumption alone. The roles of supplements include:

- Filling Nutritional Gaps: Supplements can help fill nutritional gaps in the diet. For instance, if someone doesn't consume enough fruits and vegetables, a multivitamin supplement can provide essential vitamins and minerals.

- Correcting Deficiencies: Supplements are crucial in addressing nutrient deficiencies. For example, vitamin D supplements may be recommended for those with a deficiency, especially in regions with limited sun exposure.

- Supporting Specific Health Conditions: Certain medical conditions or life stages may require specific supplements. For example, iron supplements can be essential for individuals with iron-deficiency anemia, and folic acid supplements are recommended for pregnant women to prevent birth defects.

- Enhancing Athletic Performance: Some athletes use supplements like protein powder, creatine, and branched-chain amino acids to support muscle recovery and performance.

- Promoting Bone Health: Calcium and vitamin D supplements can help maintain bone health, especially in postmenopausal women who are at risk of osteoporosis.

- Boosting Immunity: Certain vitamins and minerals, like vitamin C and zinc, are often taken to support the immune system, especially during cold and flu season.

- Managing Chronic Diseases: Supplements can be used as part of the management of chronic diseases, such as omega-3 fatty acids for heart health and coenzyme Q10 for certain heart conditions.

- Coping with Dietary Restrictions: Individuals with dietary restrictions, like vegans or those with food allergies, may take supplements to ensure they get all necessary nutrients that might be lacking in their diet.

- Antioxidant Support: Some supplements, like vitamin E and selenium, have antioxidant properties and may help reduce oxidative stress and cell damage.

- Aiding Weight Loss: Weight loss supplements can be used as part of a weight management plan, although their effectiveness and safety vary widely.

It's important to note that supplements should not be a substitute for a balanced diet. Whole foods provide a wide range of nutrients and other beneficial compounds that are not available in supplement form. Additionally, the misuse or excessive use of supplements can have negative health effects.

Before taking any supplements, it's advisable to consult with a healthcare professional, such as a doctor or registered dietitian, to determine whether they are necessary and safe for your specific needs. Furthermore, quality and safety should be considered when selecting supplements, as not all supplements on the market are regulated and proven to be effective.

Chapter 2

Fitness and Exercise Hacks

The Importance of Regular Exercise

The importance of regular exercise cannot be overstated, as it offers a wide range of physical, mental, and emotional health benefits. Incorporating regular exercise into your lifestyle can have a profound impact on your overall well-being. Key reasons why regular exercise is important:

Physical Health

Cardiovascular Health: Regular exercise strengthens the heart, improves blood circulation, and lowers the risk of heart disease, stroke, and high blood pressure.

- Weight Management: Exercise helps with weight control by burning calories and maintaining muscle mass.

- Muscle and Bone Health: It promotes muscle strength, endurance, and bone density, reducing the risk of osteoporosis.
- Improved Metabolism: Exercise supports a healthy metabolism and can help with blood sugar control, reducing the risk of type 2 diabetes.

Mental Health

- Stress Reduction: Physical activity can reduce stress levels, improve mood, and alleviate symptoms of anxiety and depression.

- Enhanced Cognitive Function: Exercise is associated with better cognitive function, memory, and increased focus.

- Better Sleep: Regular exercise can lead to improved sleep quality and duration, which is essential for mental well-being.

Emotional Well-Being

- Boosted Self-Esteem: Achieving fitness goals and feeling physically capable can boost self-esteem and confidence.

- Social Interaction: Group fitness activities and team sports provide social interaction, support, and a sense of belonging.

- Mood Regulation: Exercise triggers the release of endorphins, which can create feelings of happiness and contentment.

Disease Prevention and Management

- Exercise can help prevent or manage a wide range of health conditions, including obesity, heart disease, certain cancers, and chronic diseases like arthritis.

- Longevity: Regular exercise is linked to a longer and healthier life. It reduces the risk of premature death from various causes.

- Energy and Vitality: Exercise can increase overall energy levels and reduce feelings of fatigue. It promotes vitality and an active lifestyle.

- Better Quality of Life: Physical fitness enhances the ability to perform daily tasks, maintain independence, and engage in activities you enjoy.

- Immune System Support: Moderate exercise can boost the immune system, helping the body fight off infections and illnesses.

- Weight Loss and Maintenance: Exercise is a key component of successful weight loss and weight maintenance, especially when combined with a balanced diet.

- Lifestyle Balance: Regular exercise encourages a balanced lifestyle, helping individuals manage the demands of work, family, and personal well-being.

It's important to remember that the benefits of exercise are not limited to high-intensity workouts. Even moderate-intensity activities like walking, swimming, and gardening can contribute to improved health. The key is to find activities you enjoy and make them a regular part of your routine. Before starting a new exercise program, it's advisable to consult with a healthcare professional, especially if you have any underlying health concerns or conditions.

Cardiovascular Health

Cardiovascular health, also known as heart health, refers to the overall well-being of the heart and blood vessels. It is a critical aspect of overall health because the cardiovascular system plays a central role in supplying oxygen and nutrients to all the body's cells. Maintaining good cardiovascular health is vital for preventing heart disease and related conditions. These are key aspects of cardiovascular health:

- Heart Health: A healthy heart is the cornerstone of cardiovascular health. It involves the efficient pumping of blood throughout the body, providing oxygen and nutrients to organs and tissues.

- Blood Vessels: Healthy blood vessels are essential for proper blood flow. This includes arteries that carry oxygen-rich blood away from the heart, veins that return oxygen-poor blood to the heart, and smaller vessels called capillaries that exchange nutrients and oxygen with tissues.

- Cholesterol Levels: Maintaining healthy cholesterol levels is crucial for cardiovascular health. High levels of low-density lipoprotein (LDL) cholesterol can increase the risk of plaque buildup in arteries, while high-density lipoprotein (HDL) cholesterol is considered protective.

- Blood Pressure: Proper blood pressure regulation is vital. High blood pressure (hypertension) can strain the heart and blood vessels, increasing the risk of heart disease.

- Heart Rate: A normal heart rate reflects the heart's efficiency. Resting heart rate and heart rate variability can provide insights into cardiovascular health.

- Physical Activity: Regular exercise strengthens the heart and improves cardiovascular health. It helps lower blood pressure, reduce cholesterol, and maintain a healthy weight.

- Diet: A heart-healthy diet emphasizes whole foods, fruits, vegetables, whole grains, lean proteins, and healthy fats while minimizing saturated and trans fats, salt, and added sugars.

- Avoiding Smoking: Smoking is a significant risk factor for cardiovascular disease. Quitting smoking can lead to immediate and long-term improvements in heart health.

- Diabetes Management: Diabetes can increase the risk of heart disease. Proper management of blood sugar levels is important for cardiovascular health.

- Stress Management: Chronic stress can contribute to heart disease. Stress management techniques, such as meditation and relaxation exercises, can support cardiovascular health.

- Regular Check-Ups: Routine medical check-ups are essential for monitoring cardiovascular health, detecting risk factors early, and receiving guidance on maintaining heart health.

- Medications: In some cases, medications are prescribed to manage conditions like high blood pressure or cholesterol levels.

Maintaining good cardiovascular health is a lifelong endeavor. Making healthy lifestyle choices, such as eating a balanced diet, staying physically active, and avoiding smoking, can significantly reduce the risk of heart disease. Additionally, regular check-ups with a healthcare provider can help identify and address risk factors and provide personalized guidance on maintaining cardiovascular health.

Strength training, also known as resistance training or weight training, is a form of exercise that focuses on building and maintaining muscle strength and endurance. It plays a significant role in promoting longevity and overall health. Below is why strength training is important for longevity:

- Muscle Mass Preservation: As we age, we naturally lose muscle mass and strength, a process known as sarcopenia. Strength training helps preserve and even increase muscle mass, which is essential for maintaining mobility, balance, and independence in later years.

- Bone Health: Strength training promotes bone density and can help prevent osteoporosis, a condition characterized by weak and brittle bones. Strong muscles also provide better support for bones and reduce the risk of fractures.

- Metabolism and Weight Management: Muscle tissue burns more calories at rest than fat tissue. Building and maintaining muscle through strength training can boost metabolism, making it easier to manage and maintain a healthy weight.

- Joint Health: Strong muscles provide better support and protection to the joints. This can help reduce the risk of joint-related issues and pain, such as arthritis.

- Functional Fitness: Strength training enhances functional fitness, making everyday tasks, such as carrying groceries, climbing stairs, or getting up from a chair, easier and more manageable, promoting independence.

- Heart Health: Strength training can contribute to improved heart health by reducing risk factors such as high blood pressure and insulin resistance.

- Hormone Regulation: Strength training has been shown to positively influence hormone levels, including increasing the production of growth hormone and testosterone, both of which play a role in cellular repair and longevity.

- Balance and Fall Prevention: Building leg and core strength through strength training can improve balance and coordination, reducing the risk of falls and injuries, which can have serious consequences in older adults.

- Cognitive Function: Emerging research suggests a link between strength training and improved cognitive function. It may help protect against cognitive decline and neurodegenerative diseases.

- Psychological Well-Being: Strength training can boost self-esteem and self-confidence. It's also a great stress reliever and can help combat symptoms of depression and anxiety.

To reap the benefits of strength training for longevity, it's important to include it as part of a well-rounded fitness routine. This can be achieved through various methods, including lifting weights, bodyweight exercises, resistance bands, and other forms of resistance training.

A well-structured and progressive strength training program, combined with cardiovascular exercise and flexibility training, can contribute to a longer and healthier life. Before starting a new exercise program, it's advisable to consult with a healthcare professional or a certified fitness trainer to ensure that the program is safe and appropriate for your individual needs and goals.

Flexibility and Mobility

Flexibility and mobility are important components of physical fitness that contribute to overall well-being and functional independence. While they are closely related, they are not the same:

Flexibility

- Definition: Flexibility refers to the range of motion in a joint or group of joints. It's the ability of muscles, tendons, and ligaments to stretch and lengthen without causing injury.

- Benefits: Improved flexibility can enhance posture, reduce the risk of muscle strains and injuries, and make everyday movements easier. It can also help prevent or alleviate joint and muscle pain.

- Activities: Stretching exercises, such as static stretching, dynamic stretching, and yoga, are effective for improving flexibility.

Mobility

Mobility refers to the ability of a joint to move freely through its full range of motion. It involves both the joint's flexibility and the strength of the muscles surrounding it.

- Benefits: Good joint mobility supports functional movements, such as walking, lifting, and reaching. It also helps prevent joint stiffness and reduces the risk of injury.

- Activities: Activities that enhance mobility include dynamic warm-up exercises, joint mobility drills, and exercises that mimic everyday movements.

The importance of flexibility and mobility for overall health and longevity is significant. This is why they matter:

- Preventing Injuries: Flexible and mobile joints and muscles are less prone to strains, sprains, and other injuries, especially as you age.

- Maintaining Functional Independence: Flexibility and mobility are essential for performing daily activities, from tying shoelaces to reaching items on high shelves.

- Pain Reduction: Improving flexibility and mobility can alleviate joint and muscle pain, making movement more comfortable.

- Posture Improvement: Enhanced flexibility and mobility can support better posture, reducing the risk of musculoskeletal issues and back pain.

- Enhancing Athletic Performance: For athletes and those engaged in sports and physical activities, flexibility and mobility can improve performance and reduce the risk of overuse injuries.

- Stress Reduction: Stretching and mobility exercises can be relaxing and reduce stress, contributing to better mental and emotional well-being.

To improve flexibility and mobility, consider incorporating stretching and mobility exercises into your daily routine. Focus on stretching all major muscle groups and pay attention to areas that tend to be tight or stiff. It's important to warm up before stretching to reduce the risk of injury. Additionally, if you have specific concerns or limitations, it's advisable to consult with a healthcare professional or a qualified fitness trainer who can provide guidance on safe and effective stretching and mobility exercises tailored to your individual needs.

Mind-Body Connection

The mind-body connection is a holistic concept that emphasizes the interrelationship between mental and emotional well-being and physical health. It means that our thoughts, emotions, and mental state can profoundly impact our physical health and vice versa. This is why a closer look at the mind-body connection and why it's important for overall well-being and longevity:

Physical Health and Well-Being

The mind-body connection recognizes that psychological factors, such as stress, anxiety, and depression, can have a significant impact on physical health.

Chronic stress, for example, can lead to a variety of health problems, including cardiovascular issues, digestive disorders, and weakened immune function.

Pain Perception and Management

Our thoughts and emotions can influence our perception of pain. Techniques like mindfulness and relaxation can help individuals manage pain more effectively and reduce reliance on medication.

Immune Function

A positive mental state and emotional well-being can support a robust immune system. Stress and negative emotions can weaken immune function, making individuals more susceptible to illness.

Chronic Disease Prevention and Management

Mental and emotional well-being plays a role in preventing and managing chronic diseases. Practices like meditation and stress reduction can be beneficial for individuals dealing with conditions such as heart disease, diabetes, and autoimmune disorders.

Cognitive Function

The mind-body connection acknowledges the influence of emotional health on cognitive function. Chronic stress, for instance, can impair memory and decision-making abilities.

Stress Reduction and Resilience

Techniques that promote the mind-body connection, such as mindfulness and meditation, are effective for reducing stress and enhancing resilience. These practices can help individuals cope with life's challenges and reduce the harmful effects of stress on health.

Quality of Life and Longevity

A strong mind-body connection contributes to an improved quality of life and may enhance longevity. Emotional well-being, social connections, and a positive outlook on life are linked to a longer and healthier life.

Holistic Health Approach

A holistic approach to health, which considers the mind, body, and spirit as interconnected, encourages individuals to take responsibility for their overall well-being and make choices that support their mental, emotional, and physical health.

To enhance the mind-body connection and promote well-being, consider incorporating practices such as mindfulness meditation, yoga, deep breathing exercises, and relaxation techniques into your daily routine. Additionally, seeking support from mental health professionals, like psychologists or counselors, can provide valuable guidance in managing emotional and psychological well-being. Understanding and nurturing the mind-body connection can lead to a more balanced and fulfilling life.

Chapter 3

Mental and Emotional Well-Being Hacks

Mental and emotional well-being refers to the state of being mentally and emotionally healthy, with a positive sense of self, the ability to manage life's challenges, and the capacity to maintain fulfilling relationships. It is a fundamental aspect of overall well-being and quality of life. Having a positive self-image involves self-acceptance, self-confidence, and self-esteem. It's about valuing and respecting yourself as a unique individual.

Emotional well-being includes the ability to recognize, understand, and manage one's emotions effectively. This involves coping with stress, anger, sadness, and other emotions in a healthy way. Resilience is the capacity to bounce back from adversity, adapt to change, and handle life's challenges. It's a key component of emotional well-being.

Effective stress management techniques are essential for mental and emotional well-being. This includes practices like relaxation, mindfulness, and time management. Healthy and fulfilling relationships contribute to emotional well-being. Building and maintaining strong connections with friends, family, and loved ones is vital.

Mindfulness practices, such as meditation, and self-care routines are beneficial for emotional well-being. They promote self-awareness, inner peace, and relaxation. Maintaining a positive outlook on life, even in the face of challenges, is a hallmark of mental and emotional well-being. It can enhance overall life satisfaction.

Being able to communicate your thoughts, feelings, and needs with others fosters healthy relationships and supports emotional well-being. Psychological resilience involves the ability to overcome traumatic experiences and develop strength and growth from adversity.

Effective coping strategies are important for managing difficult situations and emotions. These strategies can include problem-solving, seeking support, and engaging in hobbies and activities that bring joy.

The importance of mental and emotional well-being cannot be overstated:

- It contributes to a higher quality of life and greater life satisfaction.
- It supports physical health, as positive emotions and low stress levels are associated with better physical health outcomes.
- Mental and emotional well-being can improve cognitive function and creativity.
- It reduces the risk of mental health disorders, such as anxiety and depression.
- Strong emotional and psychological health enables individuals to face life's challenges with resilience and adaptability.

Practices like mindfulness, meditation, therapy, social support, and self-care routines can all be valuable tools in enhancing mental and emotional well-being. Additionally, reaching out to mental health professionals when needed is important for managing and improving one's emotional and psychological health.

Stress Management

Stress management refers to a set of techniques and strategies used to cope with and reduce the negative effects of stress on physical, mental, and emotional well-being. In today's fast-paced world, managing stress is essential for maintaining good health and overall quality of life. These are some effective stress management strategies:

Identify Stressors

Begin by identifying the sources of your stress. Recognizing what is causing your stress can be the first step in addressing it.

Healthy Lifestyle Habits

- Regular Exercise: Physical activity can reduce stress and boost mood. Aim for at least 30 minutes of moderate exercise most days of the week.
- Balanced Diet: Proper nutrition supports stress management. Avoid excessive caffeine and sugar, which can exacerbate stress.

Sleep

Prioritize good sleep hygiene. A consistent sleep schedule and a relaxing bedtime routine can improve sleep quality and reduce stress.

Mindfulness and Relaxation Techniques

- Meditation: Mindfulness meditation can help calm the mind and reduce stress. Even just a few minutes of meditation daily can be effective.

- Deep Breathing: Deep, slow breathing exercises can reduce the physical symptoms of stress, such as rapid heart rate and shallow breathing.
- Progressive Muscle Relaxation: This technique involves systematically tensing and relaxing muscle groups to reduce physical tension.

Time Management

- Organize your tasks and prioritize them. Break tasks into manageable segments, and set realistic goals.
- Learn to say no to additional commitments when you're already feeling overwhelmed.

Social Support

- Talk to friends, family, or a counselor about your stressors and feelings. Social support is a powerful stress reducer.

Maintain a Positive Outlook

- Develop a positive attitude. Reframe negative thoughts into more positive and constructive ones.
- Practice gratitude to focus on the positive aspects of your life.

Limit Screen Time

- Reducing exposure to news and social media, especially if it's a source of stress, can be beneficial for stress management.

Seek Professional Help

- If stress becomes overwhelming or leads to symptoms of anxiety or depression, consider seeking the guidance of a mental health professional.

Self-Care

- Prioritize self-care activities that bring you joy, whether it's reading, spending time in nature, pursuing hobbies, or taking a relaxing bath.

Set Boundaries

Establish clear boundaries in your personal and professional life to prevent burnout and reduce stress.

Time in Nature

Spending time outdoors and connecting with nature can have a calming and stress-reducing effect.

It's important to remember that stress is a normal part of life, and some level of stress can even be motivating. However, chronic or excessive stress can lead to health problems. Effective stress management techniques can help you reduce the negative impact of stress on your life and improve your overall well-being. Experiment with different strategies to find what works best for you, and don't hesitate to seek professional help if you're struggling to manage stress on your own.

Social Connections

Social connections, also known as social relationships or social support, are vital for human well-being and longevity. Having meaningful relationships and connections with others can have a profound impact on your physical, mental, and emotional health. These are some of the reasons why social connections are important:

Mental and Emotional Well-Being

- Social connections provide emotional support, which can help reduce stress, anxiety, and depression.
- Interacting with others can boost mood, reduce feelings of loneliness, and increase feelings of happiness and well-being.

Coping with Life's Challenges

- Social support can help individuals cope with challenging life events, such as the loss of a loved one, illness, or job-related stress.
- Talking to friends and loved ones about your problems can provide comfort and perspective.

Physical Health

- Strong social connections are associated with better physical health and increased longevity.

- Having a social network can lead to healthier lifestyle choices, such as regular exercise and balanced nutrition.

Reduced Risk of Chronic Diseases

- Social isolation is linked to an increased risk of chronic diseases, such as heart disease, hypertension, and obesity.
- Engaging in social activities and maintaining relationships can reduce these risks.

Cognitive Function

- Social interactions stimulate cognitive function and can improve memory and problem-solving skills.

- Engaging in social activities and conversations can support cognitive health as you age.

Increased Resilience

- Social connections enhance resilience by providing a sense of belonging and a safety net during difficult times.
- Feeling supported by others can help individuals bounce back from adversity.

Strengthened Immune System

- Social connections have been associated with a stronger immune system, helping the body fight off infections and illnesses more effectively.

Longevity

- Having strong social connections is one of the factors associated with a longer life. A robust social network can provide motivation, purpose, and a sense of fulfillment.

Sense of Belonging

- Social connections foster a sense of belonging, which is a fundamental human need. Feeling part of a community or group can increase self-esteem and life satisfaction.

Lifelong Learning

- Engaging in social activities, such as conversations and group activities, provides opportunities for learning and personal growth.

To cultivate and maintain social connections, consider the following:

- Spend time with family and friends regularly, whether in person or virtually.
- Join clubs, organizations, or community groups that align with your interests.
- Volunteer for a cause you care about to meet like-minded individuals.
- Practice active listening and effective communication to build stronger connections with others.
- Nurture existing relationships and make an effort to reach out and stay connected.
- Seek professional help or counseling if you're struggling with feelings of loneliness or social isolation.

Building and maintaining social connections is a lifelong endeavor that requires effort and commitment. The benefits of a strong social network extend to all areas of life and contribute to a happier, healthier, and longer life.

Social Connections

Social connections, often referred to as social relationships or social networks, are the bonds and interactions we have with other individuals, whether they are family members, friends, colleagues, or acquaintances. These connections play a vital role in our well-being and overall quality of life. Let's take a closer look at the importance of social connections:

Emotional Support

Social connections provide a support system that can help individuals cope with stress, adversity, and emotional challenges. Having someone to confide in and share your feelings with can be comforting and therapeutic.

Mental Health

Strong social connections are associated with improved mental health. They can help reduce feelings of loneliness, depression, and anxiety, and promote overall psychological well-being.

Physical Health

Social interactions can have a positive impact on physical health. People with robust social networks tend to live longer and have better physical health outcomes. Social support can contribute to healthy lifestyle choices and reduce the risk of chronic diseases.

Quality of Life

Social connections enhance the quality of life by providing a sense of belonging, meaning, and fulfillment. They can add joy and purpose to daily life.

Cognitive Function

Engaging in conversations and activities with others stimulates cognitive function. It can improve memory, problem-solving skills, and overall brain health.

Resilience

Social connections can increase resilience in the face of life's challenges. Knowing you have a network of people who care about you can provide the strength to bounce back from adversity.

Happiness

Interacting with others and building meaningful relationships can boost mood and increase feelings of happiness and contentment.

Reduced Risk of Loneliness

Social connections are a powerful antidote to loneliness, which can have detrimental effects on mental and physical health. Loneliness is more likely to occur in the absence of meaningful social connections.

Sense of Belonging

Being part of a social group, whether it's a family, circle of friends, or community, fulfills the fundamental human need for a sense of belonging.

Personal Growth

Social connections provide opportunities for personal growth, learning, and development. Interactions with others expose us to new ideas, perspectives, and experiences.

The following will help to foster and strengthen social connections:

- Make time for regular interactions with family and friends.
- Join clubs, organizations, or community groups that align with your interests and values.
- Volunteer for causes you care about to meet like-minded individuals.
- Practice active listening and effective communication to build deeper connections with others.
- Reconnect with old friends or reach out to acquaintances to expand your social network.

While social connections are essential for overall well-being, it's also important to maintain a balance that aligns with your personal preferences and needs. Some people thrive in large social circles, while others prefer smaller, close-knit relationships. Ultimately, the quality of connections matters more than the quantity. Cultivating and nurturing meaningful relationships can have a profound and lasting impact on your life.

The power of positive thinking refers to the influence of a positive mindset on an individual's outlook, emotions, actions, and overall well-being. Positive thinking is characterized by an optimistic and constructive attitude, where individuals focus on solutions, opportunities, and the brighter side of situations. This is why the power of positive thinking is significant:

Emotional Well-Being

- Positive thinking can lead to increased feelings of happiness, contentment, and emotional well-being. It reduces stress, anxiety, and symptoms of depression.

Resilience

- A positive mindset fosters resilience, helping individuals bounce back from setbacks and adversity more effectively.

Improved Health

- There's evidence to suggest that positive thinking is associated with better physical health. It can lead to lower blood pressure, enhanced immune function, and a reduced risk of chronic diseases.

Stress Reduction

- Positive thinking reduces the impact of stress. It helps individuals approach challenges with a more calm and constructive attitude.

Problem-Solving

- Positive thinkers tend to be more effective problem solvers. They approach issues with a solution-oriented mindset.

Optimism

- A positive mindset fosters optimism, which can lead to increased motivation, goal-setting, and achievement.

Stronger Relationships

- Positive individuals often find it easier to build and maintain strong and fulfilling relationships. They are more enjoyable to be around and are better at providing emotional support to others.

Personal Growth

- Positive thinkers are more open to personal growth and learning. They view challenges as opportunities for self-improvement.

Boosted Self-Esteem

- A positive mindset enhances self-esteem and self-confidence, which can lead to greater life satisfaction.

Increased Energy and Productivity

- Positive thinking can boost energy levels, increasing motivation and productivity.

These will help to embrace the power of positive thinking:

- Cultivate self-awareness by monitoring your thoughts and replacing negative self-talk with more constructive language.
- Focus on gratitude by regularly reflecting on the positive aspects of your life and the things you are thankful for.
- Surround yourself with positive influences, such as supportive friends and inspirational content.
- Practice mindfulness and meditation to stay present, reduce rumination, and improve overall mental well-being.
- Set achievable goals and stay committed to them. Break goals into smaller, manageable steps and celebrate your progress.
- Recognize that setbacks and challenges are a part of life. Approach them with a problem-solving mindset, and view them as opportunities for growth.

While positive thinking is powerful, it's vital to maintain a balanced perspective. It's not about denying or ignoring negative aspects of life but rather focusing on the positive in parallel with addressing challenges. Positive thinking can be cultivated and developed over time through practice and conscious effort, leading to a happier and more fulfilling life.

Chapter 4

Sleep and Rest Hacks

Sleep and rest are essential components of overall health and well-being. While they are related, they serve slightly different purposes and occur in various context. Sleep is a naturally occurring state of unconsciousness during which the brain and body undergo essential processes for physical and mental restoration. It is characterized by distinct stages and cycles, including non-rapid eye movement (NREM) and rapid eye movement (REM) sleep.

Functions of Sleep: Sleep plays several critical roles, including:

- Physical Restoration: During deep NREM sleep, the body repairs and regenerates tissues, muscles, and the immune system.
- Memory Consolidation: REM sleep is associated with memory consolidation, helping to store and organize information.
- Emotional Processing: Sleep aids in processing and regulating emotions, which is essential for mental well-being.
- Hormone Regulation: Sleep is crucial for regulating hormones, including those involved in stress, growth, and appetite.

Circadian Rhythms

- Sleep is influenced by the body's internal clock, known as circadian rhythms, which regulate the sleep-wake cycle. These rhythms are tied to the 24-hour day-night cycle and influence the timing of sleep.

Rest

Rest is a broader concept that includes activities and moments of relaxation or inactivity that allow the body and mind to recover and recharge. While sleep is a form of rest, rest can also occur when awake.

Types of Rest: Rest can take various forms, such as:

- Physical Rest: Allowing the body to recover from physical exertion and strain.
- Mental Rest: Giving the mind a break from cognitive tasks and stress.
- Emotional Rest: Focusing on activities that promote emotional well-being and relaxation.
- Sensory Rest: Reducing sensory input to rest the senses, such as spending time in quiet or nature.

Importance of Rest

Rest is essential to recharge and maintain energy levels, reduce stress, and prevent burnout.

- Taking breaks, practicing relaxation techniques, and enjoying leisure activities contribute to overall well-being.

Balancing Sleep and Rest: Both sleep and rest are crucial for health and vitality. Striking a balance between getting enough quality sleep and incorporating periods of rest during the day is key to maintaining well-being.

Sleep Hygiene:

- Establishing good sleep hygiene practices can promote restful sleep. This includes maintaining a consistent sleep schedule, creating a comfortable sleep environment, and avoiding stimulating activities before bedtime.

Stress Management

- Effective stress management is essential for quality rest and sleep. Techniques like relaxation, mindfulness, and time management can support both.

Mind-Body Connection:

- The mind and body are interconnected when it comes to sleep and rest. Reducing mental and emotional stress can lead to better sleep, and quality sleep contributes to mental and emotional well-being.

Striving for a balance between restful sleep and periods of rest during the day can significantly enhance overall well-being. Prioritizing sleep and incorporating moments of rest into your daily routine can lead to improved physical, mental, and emotional health, allowing you to perform at your best and enjoy life to the fullest.

The science of sleep, also known as sleep medicine, is a multidisciplinary field that studies various aspects of sleep, including its stages, functions, disorders, and the impact of sleep on physical and mental health. Sleep is a fundamental physiological process that is crucial for overall well-being. These are key aspects of the science of sleep:

Stages of Sleep

- Sleep is divided into two main categories: non-rapid eye movement (NREM) sleep and rapid eye movement (REM) sleep. NREM sleep is further divided into three stages, each characterized by distinct brain wave patterns.

Sleep Cycle

- Sleep occurs in cycles, typically lasting about 90 minutes. Each cycle consists of NREM and REM stages. As the night progresses, the proportion of REM sleep increases.

Functions of Sleep

- Sleep serves multiple vital functions, including physical and mental restoration, memory consolidation, and emotional processing. It also helps regulate various physiological processes, such as hormone release and immune function.

Circadian Rhythms

- The body's internal clock, known as the circadian rhythm, regulates the sleep-wake cycle. It is influenced by external factors like light and darkness and plays a crucial role in maintaining a regular sleep pattern.

Sleep Disorders

- Sleep disorders are conditions that disrupt normal sleep patterns and can have significant health consequences. Examples include insomnia, sleep apnea, narcolepsy, and restless leg syndrome.

Sleep and Health

- Sleep is closely linked to overall health. Chronic sleep deprivation is associated with an increased risk of various health issues, including cardiovascular disease, diabetes, obesity, and mental health disorders.

Sleep Hygiene

- Sleep hygiene practices involve creating a sleep-conducive environment and adopting habits that promote healthy sleep. This includes maintaining a regular sleep schedule, avoiding stimulants before bedtime, and ensuring a comfortable sleep environment.

Sleep Technology

- Advancements in technology have led to the development of sleep-tracking devices and apps that monitor sleep patterns and provide insights into sleep quality. These can be useful for individuals looking to improve their sleep.

Treatment and Interventions

- The field of sleep medicine offers various treatments and interventions for sleep disorders. These may include behavioral therapies, lifestyle modifications, medication, and the use of medical devices, such as continuous positive airway pressure (CPAP) machines for sleep apnea.

Research and Ongoing Studies

- Ongoing research in the science of sleep continues to deepen our understanding of sleep and its impact on health. Researchers investigate areas like sleep genetics, the relationship between sleep and neurodegenerative diseases, and innovative treatments for sleep disorders.

Understanding the science of sleep is essential for maintaining good health and well-being. If you're experiencing persistent sleep problems or suspect a sleep disorder, it's advisable to consult with a healthcare professional or a sleep specialist who can provide guidance, diagnosis, and treatment options tailored to your specific needs. Quality sleep is a cornerstone of physical and mental health, and it's worth prioritizing for a better quality of life.

Creating a Sleep-Friendly Environment

Creating a sleep-friendly environment, also known as practicing good sleep hygiene, is essential for getting quality sleep and promoting overall well-being. Tips for making your sleep environment conducive to restful sleep:

Quietness

- Minimize noise disturbances by using earplugs or a white noise machine if needed. Consider noise-canceling headphones if you live in a noisy area.

Comfortable Bed and Bedding

- Invest in a comfortable mattress and pillows that provide adequate support. Make sure your bedding, including sheets and blankets, is suitable for your climate and personal comfort preferences.

Cool Temperature

- Keep the bedroom at a cool, comfortable temperature. Most people sleep best in a slightly cooler room, typically between 60-67°F (15-20°C).

Clutter-Free Space

- A cluttered bedroom can contribute to a cluttered mind. Keep your sleep environment tidy and free of distractions.

Reduce Screens

- Avoid electronic devices, such as smartphones, tablets, and TVs, at least an hour before bedtime. The blue light emitted from screens can interfere with your body's production of melatonin, a sleep-inducing hormone.

Soft Lighting

- Use soft, dim lighting in the evening to signal to your body that it's time to wind down. Consider using low-wattage bulbs or a bedside lamp with warm light.

Bedtime Routine

- Establish a calming bedtime routine to signal to your body that it's time to sleep. This can include activities like reading a book, taking a warm bath, or practicing relaxation techniques.

Limit Caffeine and Alcohol

Avoid caffeine and alcohol in the hours leading up to bedtime. These substances can interfere with your ability to fall asleep and stay asleep.

Regular Sleep Schedule

- Go to bed and wake up at the same time every day, even on weekends. This helps regulate your body's internal clock and improve the quality of your sleep.

Limit Liquid Intake Before Bed

- To avoid waking up during the night to use the bathroom, reduce your liquid intake in the hours before bedtime.

Avoid Heavy Meals Before Bed

- Large, heavy meals shortly before bedtime can disrupt sleep. Try to eat at least a couple of hours before going to bed.

Limit Daytime Naps

- If you take daytime naps, keep them short (20-30 minutes) and not too close to bedtime. Long or late naps can interfere with nighttime sleep.

Create a Relaxing Atmosphere

- Incorporate soothing elements into your bedroom decor, such as calming colors and comfortable furnishings.

Manage Stress

- Practice stress-reduction techniques like meditation, deep breathing, or progressive muscle relaxation to calm your mind before sleep.

Keep Electronics Out of the Bedroom

- Avoid using your bedroom for work or watching TV. Reserve it primarily for sleep and intimacy.

Remember that the sleep environment is highly individual, and what works best for one person may not work for another. Experiment with these tips to create a sleep-friendly space that aligns with your personal preferences and needs. Quality sleep is a cornerstone of good health and well-being, and optimizing your sleep environment can help you achieve it.

Sleep Hygiene Habits

Sleep hygiene habits are practices and behaviors that promote good sleep and healthy sleep patterns. Incorporating these habits into your daily routine can help you get better-quality sleep, improve your overall well-being, and reduce the risk of sleep disorders. These are some key sleep hygiene habits to consider:

Establish a Consistent Sleep Schedule: Go to bed and wake up at the same time every day, even on weekends. This helps regulate your body's internal clock.

Create a Comfortable Sleep Environment
- Make sure your bedroom is conducive to sleep by keeping it dark, quiet, and at a comfortable temperature.
- Invest in a comfortable mattress and pillows that provide the support you need.

Limit Exposure to Screens Before Bed: Avoid electronic devices, such as smartphones, tablets, and TVs, at least an hour before bedtime. The blue light emitted from screens can disrupt your sleep-wake cycle.

Establish a Relaxing Bedtime Routine: Engage in calming activities before bed, such as reading a book, taking a warm bath, or practicing relaxation techniques like deep breathing.

Limit Caffeine and Alcohol Intake: Avoid consuming caffeine and alcohol in the hours leading up to bedtime, as they can interfere with your ability to fall asleep and stay asleep.

Limit Liquid Intake Before Bed: Reduce your fluid intake in the evening to avoid waking up during the night to use the bathroom.

Avoid Heavy Meals Before Bed: Refrain from consuming large, heavy meals right before bedtime. Eating at least a couple of hours before sleep can improve sleep quality.

Exercise Regularly: Regular physical activity can improve sleep, but try to complete your workout at least a few hours before bedtime to allow your body time to wind down.

Manage Stress: Practice stress-reduction techniques like meditation, progressive muscle relaxation, or mindfulness to help calm your mind before sleep.

Limit Daytime Naps: If you take daytime naps, keep them short (20-30 minutes) and not too close to bedtime. Long or late naps can interfere with nighttime sleep.

Reserve the Bedroom for Sleep and Intimacy: Avoid using your bedroom for work or watching TV. Reserve it primarily for sleep and intimate activities.

Expose Yourself to Natural Light: Spend time outdoors during the day to regulate your circadian rhythm. Natural light exposure during the morning can help signal to your body that it's time to be awake.

Limit Clock Watching: Constantly checking the time during the night can create anxiety about not sleeping. Consider removing the clock from your line of sight or covering it.

Engage in Relaxation Activities: Relaxation techniques like meditation, progressive muscle relaxation, and deep breathing exercises can help you unwind and prepare your body for sleep.

Consult a Healthcare Professional:

If you have persistent sleep problems or suspect a sleep disorder, consult a healthcare professional or sleep specialist for evaluation and guidance.

Consistently practicing good sleep hygiene habits can significantly improve the quality of your sleep and contribute to better physical and mental health. While it may take time to establish these habits, the benefits of restful sleep are well worth the effort.

Napping for Longevity

Napping can have both positive and negative effects on longevity, depending on how and when it's done. Here's a closer look at the relationship between napping and longevity:

Positive Aspects of Napping for Longevity:

1. Cognitive Benefits: Short naps, typically lasting 20-30 minutes, can boost cognitive function, improve alertness, and enhance memory. These benefits can contribute to overall mental well-being as you age.

2. Stress Reduction: A brief nap can help reduce stress and promote relaxation, which is important for heart health and overall longevity.

3. Improved Mood: Napping can elevate mood and help alleviate feelings of irritability and fatigue, enhancing emotional well-being.

Negative Aspects of Excessive or Long Napping:

1. Sleep Disruption: Long or irregular napping during the day can disrupt nighttime sleep patterns. This may lead to sleep disorders, such as insomnia, which can negatively impact overall health and longevity.

2. Risk of Chronic Diseases: Some studies suggest that excessive daytime napping (longer than an hour) may be associated with an increased risk of chronic diseases, such as heart disease and diabetes.

3. Daytime Sleepiness: Extended napping during the day can lead to increased daytime sleepiness, which may impact overall productivity and quality of life.

4. Circadian Rhythm Disruption: Irregular or long naps can disrupt your body's natural circadian rhythms, which play a crucial role in maintaining a regular sleep-wake cycle. Disrupted circadian rhythms are associated with a higher risk of health problems.

Tips for Napping with Longevity in Mind:

- If you choose to nap, aim for a short nap of 20-30 minutes. This can help improve alertness and cognitive function without interfering with nighttime sleep.
- Try to nap earlier in the day to avoid disrupting your circadian rhythm. Late afternoon naps may interfere with nighttime sleep.
- Pay attention to your body's signals. If you consistently feel the need to nap during the day, it may be an indication of insufficient nighttime sleep. In this case, focus on improving nighttime sleep quality.

- If you have sleep disorders or chronic health conditions, consult with a healthcare professional for guidance on napping and sleep patterns that support your well-being and longevity.

Ultimately, the relationship between napping and longevity is complex and individualized. Short, well-timed naps can offer cognitive and emotional benefits, but excessive or poorly timed napping can have negative consequences. It's essential to find a balance that works for you and supports your overall health and longevity goals.

Managing Insomnia

Managing insomnia involves adopting healthy sleep habits and making lifestyle changes to improve the quality and quantity of your sleep. If you're struggling with insomnia, consider the following strategies to help manage and overcome it:

1. Establish a Consistent Sleep Schedule: Go to bed and wake up at the same time every day, even on weekends. This helps regulate your body's internal clock and improve sleep quality.

2. Create a Comfortable Sleep Environment: Ensure your bedroom is dark, quiet, and at a comfortable temperature. Invest in a good mattress and pillows that provide adequate support.

3. Limit Exposure to Screens Before Bed: Avoid electronic devices, such as smartphones and computers, at least an hour before bedtime. The blue light from screens can interfere with your body's melatonin production, making it harder to fall asleep.

4. Practice Relaxation Techniques: Engage in relaxation activities before bedtime, such as reading, meditation, deep breathing exercises, or progressive muscle relaxation.

5. Limit Caffeine and Alcohol Intake: Avoid consuming caffeine and alcohol in the hours leading up to bedtime, as they can disrupt your sleep.

6. Stay Active: Regular physical activity can improve sleep, but avoid vigorous exercise close to bedtime. Aim for at least 30 minutes of moderate exercise most days.

7. Watch Your Diet: Avoid heavy meals close to bedtime. Spicy or acidic foods, as well as large meals, can cause discomfort and interfere with sleep.

8. Limit Liquid Intake Before Bed: Reduce your fluid intake in the evening to prevent waking up during the night to use the bathroom.

9. Avoid Daytime Napping: If you need to nap during the day, keep it short (20-30 minutes) and not too close to bedtime.

10. Manage Stress: Stress and anxiety are common causes of insomnia. Practice stress-reduction techniques, such as meditation or mindfulness, to relax your mind before sleep.

11. Reserve the Bedroom for Sleep and Intimacy: Avoid using your bedroom for work or watching TV. Reserve it primarily for sleep and intimate activities.

12. Seek Professional Help: If your insomnia is persistent or significantly impacts your daily life, consult with a healthcare professional or sleep specialist. They can

diagnose any underlying issues and provide guidance on treatment options, including therapy or medication.

13. Cognitive Behavioral Therapy for Insomnia (CBT-I):CBT-I is a highly effective therapeutic approach for managing insomnia. It addresses the thoughts and behaviors that contribute to sleep problems and helps you develop healthy sleep habits.

14. Medication: In some cases, healthcare professionals may prescribe medication to help manage insomnia. These are typically used for short-term relief and should be used under professional guidance.

It may take time to see improvements in your sleep patterns. Be patient and persistent in implementing these strategies, and consult with a healthcare professional for personalized guidance on managing your insomnia effectively. Quality sleep is crucial for overall well-being, and addressing insomnia can have a positive impact on your physical and mental health.

Chapter 5

Lifestyle and Habits Hacks

Lifestyle and habits play a significant role in determining your overall health, well-being, and longevity. These are some key lifestyle factors and habits that can influence your quality of life:

Diet and Nutrition: Consuming a balanced and nutritious diet is essential for good health. A diet rich in fruits, vegetables, whole grains, lean proteins, and healthy fats provides essential nutrients for your body. It's also important to stay hydrated and limit the intake of processed and sugary foods.

Physical Activity: Regular exercise is crucial for maintaining physical fitness, managing weight, and reducing the risk of chronic diseases. Aim for a combination of cardiovascular exercise, strength training, and flexibility activities.

Sleep: Quality sleep is essential for physical and mental well-being. Develop good sleep habits, maintain a consistent sleep schedule, and create a comfortable sleep environment to ensure restful sleep.

Stress Management: Chronic stress can have adverse effects on your health. Incorporate stress-reduction techniques such as mindfulness, meditation, deep breathing, and hobbies to manage stress effectively.

Social Connections: Maintain meaningful relationships with friends and family. Social connections are associated with improved mental and emotional well-being, and they provide support during challenging times.

Mental and Emotional Health: Prioritize your mental and emotional health by seeking professional help when needed. Develop coping strategies, practice gratitude, and engage in activities that bring joy and relaxation.

Hydration: Staying well-hydrated is essential for various bodily functions. Drinking enough water supports digestion, circulation, and overall health.

Alcohol and Substance Use: Consume alcohol in moderation or avoid it altogether. Avoid the use of recreational drugs and limit the use of prescription medications to their intended purposes.

Tobacco Use: Quit smoking and avoid exposure to secondhand smoke. Smoking is a leading cause of preventable diseases and significantly reduces life expectancy.

Screen Time: Manage your screen time and maintain a healthy balance between technology use and offline activities. Excessive screen time, especially before bedtime, can disrupt sleep patterns.

Preventive Healthcare: Schedule regular check-ups with healthcare providers to monitor your health and catch potential issues early. Follow recommended vaccinations, screenings, and health guidelines.

Financial Health: Manage your finances responsibly to reduce stress and ensure access to healthcare and essential resources.

Environmental Impact: Make eco-friendly choices to minimize your impact on the environment. Reducing waste, conserving resources, and supporting sustainability efforts contribute to a healthier planet.

Time Management: Effective time management can help you maintain a balanced lifestyle. Prioritize your tasks and allocate time for self-care, relaxation, and personal interests.

Personal Growth: Continuously seek personal growth and learning opportunities. Engaging in lifelong learning can improve cognitive function and enhance your quality of life.

Safety and Risk Management: Take safety precautions to reduce risks related to activities such as driving, outdoor adventures, or home maintenance.

Physical Health Screenings: Regularly visit healthcare professionals for screenings and assessments relevant to your age and gender, such as mammograms, colonoscopies, or prostate exams.

It's important to note that individual needs and circumstances vary, so it's essential to tailor your lifestyle and habits to your specific health goals and challenges. Small, consistent changes in your daily routine can have a significant impact on your long-term health and well-being. Consult with healthcare professionals and experts in relevant fields to develop a personalized plan that best suits your needs and aspirations.

Quitting Smoking

Quitting smoking is one of the most beneficial decisions you can make for your health and well-being. Smoking is a leading cause of preventable diseases and significantly reduces life expectancy. If you're looking to quit smoking, below are some steps and strategies to help you on your journey:

Set a Quit Date: Choose a specific date to quit smoking. This provides a clear goal and a sense of commitment.

Understand Your Triggers: Identify situations, emotions, and activities that trigger your smoking habit. This awareness will help you develop strategies to manage these triggers.

Seek Support: Inform your friends and family about your decision to quit. Their support can be invaluable. You can also consider joining a support group or reaching out to a healthcare professional for guidance.

Nicotine Replacement Therapy (NRT): Consider using nicotine replacement therapies, such as nicotine gum, patches, or lozenges. These products can help reduce withdrawal symptoms.

Prescription Medications: Some prescription medications, like varenicline (Chantix) or bupropion (Zyban), can aid in smoking cessation. Consult a healthcare provider to determine if these medications are suitable for you.

Create a Smoke-Free Environment:
Remove cigarettes, lighters, and ashtrays from your home and car. Make it as inconvenient as possible to smoke.

Practice Stress Management: Stress is a common trigger for smoking. Develop stress-reduction techniques, such as mindfulness, meditation, deep breathing, or physical activity.

Replace Smoking with Healthy Habits: Substitute smoking with healthier activities. For example, chew sugarless gum, go for a walk, or engage in a hobby when you feel the urge to smoke.

Stay Busy: Keep yourself occupied to reduce cravings. Plan activities that keep your mind and body engaged.

Stay Positive: Maintain a positive attitude and remind yourself of the benefits of quitting, such as improved health, increased energy, and financial savings.

Anticipate Challenges: Be prepared for challenges and slip-ups. Don't get discouraged if you have a setback. Many people make multiple attempts before successfully quitting.

Celebrate Milestones: Acknowledge and reward yourself for your achievements. Whether it's a day, a week, or a month without smoking, celebrate your progress.

Get Professional Help: If you find quitting especially challenging or have concerns about withdrawal symptoms or nicotine cravings, consult a healthcare provider or addiction specialist. They can offer personalized guidance and support.

Stay Persistent: Quitting smoking can be difficult, but persistence is key. Remind yourself of your reasons for quitting and stay committed to your goal.

Consider Support Apps and Hotlines: There are several smartphone apps and hotlines that offer support, advice, and encouragement for those trying to quit smoking. Explore these resources to help you on your journey.

Remember that quitting smoking is a process, and it's okay to seek help and support along the way. Each day without smoking brings you closer to better health and an improved quality of life. Don't be discouraged by setbacks, and keep working towards your goal of being smoke-free.

Reducing Alcohol Consumption

Reducing alcohol consumption is a positive step for your overall health and well-being. If you're looking to cut back on your alcohol intake or quit drinking altogether, the following are some strategies to help you succeed:

Set Clear Goals: Define your specific goals for reducing alcohol consumption. This could include drinking less frequently, consuming smaller quantities, or quitting altogether.

Track Your Drinking: Keep a journal of your drinking habits. This will help you understand when, where, and why you drink, making it easier to identify areas for improvement.

Identify Triggers: Recognize the situations, emotions, or social pressures that lead to increased alcohol consumption. Understanding your triggers will help you develop strategies to manage them.

Seek Support: Inform your friends and family about your decision to cut back on alcohol. Their support and encouragement can be a significant motivator. Consider joining a support group or speaking with a counselor or therapist if needed.

Set Limits: Decide on specific limits for your alcohol intake. For example, you might set a daily or weekly limit on the number of drinks you'll have.

Create Alcohol-Free Days: Dedicate certain days of the week to being alcohol-free. This can help reduce overall consumption and give your body time to recover.

Learn to Say "No": Politely decline offers of alcohol when you're in situations where you'd rather not drink. You have the right to make choices that align with your goals.

Find Alternatives: Replace alcoholic beverages with non-alcoholic options. There are many non-alcoholic beverages available that can mimic the social aspect of drinking without the alcohol.

Stay Active: Engage in regular physical activity. Exercise can help reduce stress, improve mood, and take your mind off the desire to drink.

Mindfulness and Stress Management: Develop mindfulness and stress management techniques to address the emotional triggers for drinking. Practices like meditation and deep breathing can be helpful.

Remove Temptation: Rid your home of alcohol or keep it out of sight to reduce the temptation to drink.

Seek Professional Help: If you're finding it particularly challenging to reduce alcohol consumption or are experiencing withdrawal symptoms, consult a healthcare provider or addiction specialist. They can provide personalized guidance and support.

Celebrate Success: Acknowledge and celebrate your achievements in reducing alcohol consumption. Milestones, no matter how small, are worth celebrating.

Educate Yourself: Learn about the health risks associated with excessive alcohol consumption. Knowing the potential consequences can strengthen your motivation to cut back.

Plan Ahead: Before attending social events or situations where alcohol may be present, plan strategies to resist the temptation to drink. This might include bringing your non-alcoholic beverage or having a designated driver.

Note that reducing alcohol consumption is a personal journey, and it's okay to seek support and assistance along the way. Prioritizing your health and well-being is a worthy goal, and taking steps to reduce alcohol consumption is a positive move in that direction.

Avoiding Harmful Chemicals

Avoiding harmful chemicals is an important aspect of maintaining good health and overall well-being. Many harmful chemicals can be found in everyday products, foods, and environments. Here are some strategies to help you minimize your exposure to harmful chemicals:

Read Labels: Read product labels carefully, especially for cleaning supplies, personal care products, and packaged foods. Look for items with fewer chemicals and ingredients you can understand.

Choose Natural and Organic Products: Opt for natural and organic products whenever possible. These often contain fewer synthetic chemicals and are less likely to contain harmful additives.

Use Safe Cleaning Products: Choose environmentally friendly and non-toxic cleaning products for your home. Many natural cleaning solutions, such as vinegar and baking soda, can be effective alternatives.

Minimize Plastic Use: Reduce your use of plastic products, particularly those with BPA and phthalates. Use glass or stainless steel containers for food and beverages when feasible.

Eat Organic Foods: Select organic fruits and vegetables, as they are less likely to contain pesticide residues. Also, consider reducing your consumption of processed foods with artificial additives.

Filter Your Water: Invest in a water filter for your home to remove contaminants. Drinking clean, filtered water can significantly reduce exposure to harmful chemicals.

Avoid Tobacco and Secondhand Smoke: Refrain from smoking, and avoid exposure to secondhand smoke. Cigarette smoke contains numerous harmful chemicals.

Limit Alcohol Consumption: Consume alcohol in moderation or avoid it altogether. Alcohol can be a source of harmful chemicals and has health risks associated with excessive consumption.

Reduce Chemical Use in the Garden: Use natural pest control methods in your garden to minimize the need for chemical pesticides and herbicides.

Ventilate Indoor Spaces: Ensure proper ventilation in your home to reduce indoor air pollution. Use exhaust fans and open windows to allow fresh air to circulate.

Manage Household Dust: Regularly clean and dust your home to reduce the buildup of chemicals, allergens, and contaminants.

Check for Radon: Test your home for radon gas, a naturally occurring radioactive gas that can be harmful if levels are elevated.

Be Cautious with Personal Care Products: Be selective with personal care products, such as cosmetics and skincare items. Look for products without potentially harmful ingredients like parabens and phthalates.

Filter Indoor Air: Consider using air purifiers with HEPA filters to remove airborne pollutants and allergens from your indoor environment.

Stay Informed: Keep up to date with information about harmful chemicals in products, foods, and the environment. Be aware of recalls and safety alerts.

Advocate for Change: Support policies and initiatives aimed at reducing harmful chemicals in the environment. Advocate for stronger regulations and corporate responsibility.

Minimizing exposure to harmful chemicals is an ongoing process. Small changes in your lifestyle and purchasing decisions can lead to a significant reduction in your exposure to potentially harmful substances, contributing to your long-term health and well-being.

Living a Purposeful Life

Living a purposeful life is about finding meaning, direction, and fulfillment in your everyday existence. It's a journey of self-discovery and aligning your actions with your values and passions. Some steps to help you live a more purposeful life:

Self-Reflection: Spend time reflecting on your values, interests, and aspirations. What matters most to you? What brings you joy and fulfillment? Self-awareness is the first step in living purposefully.

Set Meaningful Goals: Define clear and meaningful goals that align with your values. These goals can give your life direction and purpose, whether they are related to career, relationships, personal growth, or community involvement.

Find Your Passions: Discover your passions and what excites you. Pursuing activities and hobbies that genuinely interest you can infuse your life with purpose and enthusiasm.

Contribute and Give Back: Find ways to contribute to others and your community. Acts of kindness, volunteering, or participating in charitable initiatives can provide a sense of purpose and connection to something greater than yourself.

Connect with Others: Build and nurture meaningful relationships. Connection with family, friends, and a supportive social network can enhance your sense of belonging and purpose.

Learn Continuously: Commit to lifelong learning and personal growth. Acquiring new knowledge and skills can boost your confidence and open doors to new opportunities.

Embrace Challenges: Don't shy away from challenges or setbacks. They can be valuable learning experiences that contribute to your growth and resilience.

Live Mindfully: Practice mindfulness and being present in the moment. Mindful living can help you appreciate the beauty of everyday life and find meaning in the simplest of experiences.

Maintain a Healthy Lifestyle: Taking care of your physical health through regular exercise and a balanced diet can provide you with the energy and vitality needed to pursue your purpose.

Manage Stress: Develop effective stress management techniques, such as meditation, yoga, or deep breathing, to maintain emotional well-being and stay focused on your goals.

Simplify Your Life: Streamline your life by decluttering and letting go of material possessions and commitments that no longer serve your purpose.

Stay Resilient: Cultivate resilience and the ability to bounce back from setbacks. Resilience can help you stay committed to your goals in the face of challenges.

Seek Support and Guidance: Don't be afraid to seek guidance from mentors, coaches, or therapists. They can provide valuable insights and support on your journey toward a purposeful life.

Celebrate Your Achievements: Acknowledge and celebrate your accomplishments, both big and small. Recognizing your progress can boost your motivation and satisfaction.

Give Time to Yourself: Regularly set aside time for self-care and self-reflection. This can help you recharge and stay connected with your purpose.

Stay Open to Change: Be open to evolving your purpose as you grow and change. Your sense of purpose may shift over time, and that's perfectly normal.

Living a purposeful life is a deeply personal journey. It's about discovering what truly matters to you and actively pursuing it. By following your passions, nurturing your relationships, and staying true to your values, you can lead a more fulfilling and purpose-driven life.

Chapter 6

Preventive Healthcare Hacks

It is a proactive approach to maintaining your well-being and preventing illness or health issues before they occur. Some key elements of preventive healthcare:

Regular Check-Ups

- Schedule regular health check-ups with your healthcare provider. These visits allow for early detection of health problems and provide an opportunity to discuss any concerns or questions you may have.

Vaccinations

- Stay up-to-date on recommended vaccinations and immunizations. Vaccines can protect you from a range of diseases, from the flu to tetanus and more.

Healthy Diet

- Maintain a balanced and nutritious diet. Consume a variety of fruits, vegetables, whole grains, lean proteins, and healthy fats to provide essential nutrients for your body.

Regular Physical Activity

- Incorporate regular exercise into your routine. Aim for at least 150 minutes of moderate-intensity aerobic activity or 75 minutes of vigorous-intensity aerobic activity per week, as recommended by health guidelines.

Tobacco and Alcohol

- Avoid or limit the use of tobacco and alcohol. Smoking and excessive alcohol consumption are major risk factors for various health conditions.

Screenings and Tests

- Participate in health screenings and tests appropriate for your age and risk factors. These may include blood pressure checks, cholesterol screenings, cancer screenings, and more.

Mental Health Care

- Prioritize your mental health. Seek support and counseling when needed and practice stress management techniques to maintain emotional well-being.

Maintain a Healthy Weight

- Achieve and maintain a healthy body weight. Excess weight can contribute to a range of health problems, including heart disease, diabetes, and more.

Safe Sex Practices

- Practice safe sex to protect yourself from sexually transmitted infections (STIs). Use condoms and get regular STI screenings.

Sun Protection

- Protect your skin from the sun's harmful ultraviolet (UV) rays. Use sunscreen, wear protective clothing, and avoid excessive sun exposure to reduce the risk of skin cancer.

Dental Care

- Regular dental check-ups and oral hygiene are essential for overall health. Poor oral health is linked to various medical conditions.

Eye Examination

- Don't forget about your eye health. Schedule regular eye exams to detect vision problems and eye conditions.

Preventive Medications
- Follow your healthcare provider's recommendations for preventive medications, such as aspirin for heart health or statins for cholesterol management.

Cancer Prevention
- Be aware of your family history and genetic risks for cancer. Engage in screenings and lifestyle choices that reduce your cancer risk.

Sleep Hygiene
- Develop good sleep habits and prioritize quality sleep. Sleep is essential for physical and mental well-being.

Immunizations and Travel Health
- If you plan to travel, research the health risks in the region you're visiting and get any required or recommended vaccinations and health advice.

Stay Informed
- Keep yourself informed about the latest health guidelines and recommendations. Health advice may change over time, so staying up to date is essential.

Preventive healthcare can help you enjoy a longer, healthier life by identifying potential health issues early and taking steps to reduce risks. Consult with your healthcare provider to create a personalized preventive healthcare plan that suits your age, gender, family history, and individual health needs.

Regular Health Check-ups

Regular health check-ups are an essential component of preventive healthcare. They involve routine visits to a healthcare provider to assess your overall health, screen for specific conditions, and identify potential health issues early. Here's what you can expect during a regular health check-up:

Medical History: Your healthcare provider will review your medical history, including any existing health conditions, medications you're taking, and your family's medical history.

Vital Signs: They will measure your vital signs, including blood pressure, heart rate, and temperature.

Physical Examination: A thorough physical examination is conducted to assess your overall health. This may involve checking your heart, lungs, abdomen, and other body systems.

Blood Tests: Depending on your age and risk factors, blood tests may be ordered to assess cholesterol levels, blood sugar, liver function, kidney function, and more.

Screenings: Your healthcare provider may recommend screenings based on your age and risk factors. These could include cancer screenings (e.g., mammograms, colonoscopies), bone density tests, and other specialized tests.

Immunizations: Your vaccination status will be reviewed, and any necessary vaccinations or booster shots will be administered.

Review of Medications: Your healthcare provider will assess the medications you are taking and make any necessary adjustments.

Discussion of Symptoms and Concerns: You'll have the opportunity to discuss any symptoms you've been experiencing and any concerns about your health.

Counseling: You may receive counseling on topics such as nutrition, exercise, stress management, and mental health.

Preventive Advice: Your healthcare provider will provide guidance on preventive measures, lifestyle changes, and risk reduction strategies based on your individual health profile.

Follow-Up: If any health issues or abnormalities are identified during the check-up, your provider will recommend further testing or follow-up visits.

Regular health check-ups are essential for catching potential health problems in their early stages, when they are often more manageable and treatable. The frequency of these check-ups may vary depending on your age, gender, and individual health risk factors. It's important to work with your healthcare provider to establish a check-up schedule that's appropriate for your needs. Additionally, these visits offer an opportunity to build a strong patient-provider relationship and discuss any health concerns or goals you may have.

Vaccinations and Immunizations

Vaccinations and immunizations are essential tools for preventing and protecting against a range of infectious diseases. They work by stimulating your immune system to recognize and fight specific pathogens, such as bacteria or viruses. These are key points about vaccinations and immunizations:

Types of Vaccinations: There are various types of vaccines, including:

- Routine Vaccines: Recommended for people of all ages, such as measles, mumps, rubella (MMR), and the annual flu vaccine.
- Childhood Vaccines: Essential for children to protect against diseases like polio, chickenpox, and hepatitis B.
- Adult Vaccines: Adults may require booster shots or vaccines against diseases like tetanus, diphtheria, and shingles.
- Travel Vaccines: If traveling to certain regions, you may need vaccines to protect against diseases prevalent in those areas.
- Specialty Vaccines: Some vaccines are designed for specific populations, such as healthcare workers or those with certain health conditions.

Vaccine Schedule: Vaccinations are administered according to a schedule recommended by healthcare authorities like the Centers for Disease Control and Prevention (CDC) or the World Health Organization (WHO). This schedule ensures timely protection and may include multiple doses of a vaccine.

- Herd Immunity: Widespread vaccination in a community can create herd immunity, protecting those who cannot be vaccinated, such as individuals with certain medical conditions or compromised immune systems.

Safety and Effectiveness: Vaccines undergo rigorous testing for safety and effectiveness before being approved for use. They are continuously monitored for any potential side effects.

Common Vaccines: Some common vaccines and immunizations include.

MMR Vaccine: Protects against measles, mumps, and rubella.

Flu Vaccine: Provides annual protection against seasonal influenza.

Tetanus and Diphtheria (Td) or Tetanus, Diphtheria, and Pertussis (Tdap) Vaccine: Prevents tetanus, diphtheria, and pertussis (whooping cough).

Hepatitis B Vaccine: Guards against hepatitis B, a serious liver infection.

HPV Vaccine: Prevents certain types of human papillomavirus (HPV) that can lead to cancer.

Pneumococcal Vaccine: Protects against pneumonia and other infections caused by Streptococcus pneumoniae.

Varicella (Chickenpox) Vaccine: Prevents chickenpox.

Booster Shots: Booster shots may be recommended for some vaccines to maintain protection over time or address emerging variants of a virus.

Vaccine Hesitancy: Vaccine hesitancy is a challenge in some communities. Education, awareness, and trust-building efforts are important in addressing concerns and increasing vaccine uptake.

Travel Vaccinations: Before traveling, research the health risks in your destination and consult a healthcare provider for travel-specific vaccines and health advice.

Global Immunization Efforts: Worldwide efforts are made to increase access to vaccines, especially in low- and middle-income countries, to combat infectious diseases.

Vaccinations and immunizations have made a significant impact on public health by preventing serious diseases and reducing their spread. It's important to stay informed about recommended vaccines for yourself and your family and to consult with healthcare providers for guidance on staying up-to-date with vaccinations.

Screening for Chronic Diseases

Screening for chronic diseases is an important aspect of preventive healthcare. It involves the regular evaluation and testing for specific health conditions, often before symptoms appear, with the goal of early detection and intervention. Here are some common chronic diseases for which screening is recommended:

Cancer Screening: Cancer screenings can help detect various forms of cancer early, when treatment is often more effective. Common cancer screenings include mammograms for breast cancer, Pap smears for cervical cancer, colonoscopies for colorectal cancer, and PSA tests for prostate cancer.

Cardiovascular Disease Screening: Cardiovascular disease is a leading cause of death worldwide. Screening may include blood pressure measurement, cholesterol checks, and electrocardiograms (ECGs) to assess heart health.

Diabetes Screening: Diabetes screening is important, particularly for individuals with risk factors such as obesity, family history, or high blood sugar levels. Fasting blood sugar tests or HbA1c tests are common methods for diabetes screening.

Osteoporosis Screening: Osteoporosis is a condition that weakens bones, making them more susceptible to fractures. Bone density scans (DXA) can help detect osteoporosis, especially in postmenopausal women and older adults.

Hepatitis Screening: Hepatitis B and C screenings are important for detecting viral infections that can lead to liver damage and other health issues. These tests may be recommended for those with specific risk factors.

Lung Disease Screening: For individuals with a history of smoking, lung cancer screening with low-dose CT scans is recommended to detect lung cancer at an earlier, more treatable stage.

Kidney Disease Screening: Screening for kidney disease may involve blood tests to assess kidney function. This is particularly important for individuals with diabetes, high blood pressure, or a family history of kidney disease.

Eye and Vision Screening: Regular eye exams are essential for detecting vision problems and eye conditions, such as glaucoma or age-related macular degeneration.

Chronic Infectious Disease Screening: Depending on factors like travel history and lifestyle, screenings for infectious diseases like HIV or tuberculosis may be recommended.

Mental Health Screening: Mental health screenings, such as depression and anxiety assessments, are important for identifying and addressing mental health disorders.

Oral Health Screening: Regular dental check-ups are crucial for maintaining oral health and detecting issues like gum disease or oral cancer.

Autoimmune Disease Screening: For those with a family history of autoimmune diseases, screenings or specific blood tests may be recommended.

It's important to note that screening recommendations may vary based on factors like age, gender, family history, and individual risk factors. Always consult with your healthcare provider to determine which screenings are appropriate for you. These screenings can help detect chronic diseases in their early stages, enabling timely intervention and improved outcomes.

Managing Chronic Conditions

Managing chronic conditions involves taking ongoing steps to control, mitigate, and cope with long-term health issues. These are some strategies to help effectively manage chronic conditions:

Education and Understanding: Learn about your condition. Understanding its causes, symptoms, and treatment options is essential for effective management.

Regular Medical Check-Ups: Schedule regular visits with your healthcare provider to monitor your condition, adjust treatment plans, and address any concerns.

Medication Management: If prescribed medications, take them as directed. Keep a record of your medications and adhere to your treatment plan.

Lifestyle Modifications: Make necessary changes to your lifestyle to improve your condition. This may include adopting a healthier diet, getting regular exercise, quitting smoking, or reducing stress.

Healthy Diet: Follow a balanced diet that aligns with your condition. For example, a heart-healthy diet for cardiovascular issues or a low-sodium diet for hypertension.

Physical Activity: Engage in regular physical activity that is appropriate for your condition. Exercise can help improve your overall health and control many chronic diseases.

Weight Management: Maintain a healthy weight or lose weight if necessary. Weight management can significantly impact the management of conditions like diabetes and osteoarthritis.

Stress Management: Practice stress-reduction techniques, such as meditation, yoga, or deep breathing, to manage the emotional impact of a chronic condition.

Support and Resources: Seek support from healthcare professionals, support groups, or therapists who specialize in your condition. Connecting with others who share your experiences can be helpful.

Symptom Monitoring: Keep a record of your symptoms, their severity, and any triggers. This information can be valuable for adjusting your treatment plan.

Preventive Care: Stay current with preventive care, including vaccinations and screenings, to catch and address any potential complications.

Pain Management: If your condition involves chronic pain, work with your healthcare provider to develop a pain management plan. This may include medications, physical therapy, or other interventions.

Sleep and Rest: Get enough sleep and practice good sleep hygiene. Quality sleep can have a positive impact on many chronic conditions.

Regular Monitoring: Keep track of key health metrics, such as blood pressure, blood sugar, cholesterol levels, or any other relevant indicators.

Patient Empowerment: Take an active role in managing your condition. Discuss treatment options, ask questions, and advocate for your health.

Emergency Plan: In some cases, you may need an emergency plan for flare-ups or complications of your condition. Discuss this with your healthcare provider.

Goal Setting: Set achievable health goals with your healthcare team. These goals can help motivate you and measure your progress.

Family and Caregiver Involvement: Involve your family or caregivers in your care plan. They can provide valuable support and encouragement.

Managing a chronic condition is often a lifelong journey. By taking proactive steps, adhering to treatment plans, and making healthy lifestyle choices, you can maintain a good quality of life and reduce the impact of your condition on your daily activities. Always consult with your healthcare provider for personalized guidance on managing your specific chronic condition.

Holistic Health Approach

A holistic health approach is a comprehensive approach to well-being that considers the whole person- body, mind, and spirit. It recognizes the interconnectedness of various aspects of a person's life and health. Here are key principles and components of a holistic health approach:

Body-Mind-Spirit Connection: Holistic health recognizes that the physical, mental, and spiritual aspects of a person are interconnected and influence each other.

Preventive Focus: Emphasis is placed on prevention, rather than just treating illness or symptoms. Preventive measures can include healthy lifestyle choices, stress reduction, and regular check-ups.

Individualized Care: Holistic health is highly individualized. It acknowledges that each person is unique, with specific needs and preferences.

Balanced Nutrition: A focus on balanced and nutritious eating, emphasizing whole, unprocessed foods to nourish the body and support overall health.

Physical Activity: Regular physical activity is encouraged to maintain physical health, manage stress, and support emotional well-being.

Emotional and Mental Health: Stress reduction techniques, mindfulness, and practices for managing emotional health are key components. Mental and emotional well-being is considered integral to overall health.

Alternative Therapies: Holistic health often includes complementary and alternative therapies such as acupuncture, chiropractic care, herbal medicine, and massage therapy.

Spiritual Well-Being: The nurturing of spiritual health and well-being is encouraged. This can include practices like meditation, yoga, or participation in religious or spiritual communities.

Environmental Awareness: Recognizing the impact of the environment on health and advocating for a healthy, clean, and sustainable environment.

Social and Relationship Health: The importance of healthy social connections and relationships for overall well-being is acknowledged. Positive relationships can contribute to mental and emotional health.

Life Purpose and Fulfillment: Identifying and pursuing a sense of life purpose and fulfillment is considered important. This can provide a sense of meaning and happiness.

Holistic Healthcare Providers: Holistic healthcare providers, such as naturopathic doctors or integrative medicine practitioners, often embrace these principles and offer a holistic approach to care.

Prevention of Chronic Conditions: Efforts are made to prevent chronic conditions through lifestyle choices, early detection, and interventions that promote overall health.

Patient Empowerment: Encouraging patients to actively participate in their healthcare decisions and become advocates for their own well-being.

Mindful Living: Emphasizing mindfulness in daily life, where individuals are present in the moment, reducing stress, and enhancing overall quality of life.

Quality of Life: Holistic health focuses on enhancing the quality of life, promoting well-being beyond the absence of disease.

Preventive Health Measures: Advocating for vaccinations, screenings, and preventive health measures that can protect against various diseases and conditions.

A holistic health approach recognizes that health is not solely the absence of disease but a state of overall well-being, encompassing the physical, mental, emotional, and spiritual aspects of an individual's life. It encourages individuals to take an active role in their health, make informed choices, and achieve a sense of balance and vitality in their lives.

Chapter 7

Longevity Hacks Across the Lifespan

Longevity across the lifespan refers to the goal of living a long, healthy life at every stage of one's existence. It involves adopting a holistic approach to well-being, considering various aspects of health and life satisfaction from childhood through old age. Key principles and considerations for promoting longevity across the lifespan:

Early Childhood and Adolescence:

- Childhood health habits can have a significant impact on later life. Encourage a nutritious diet, regular physical activity, and emotional well-being from a young age.

Education:

- Access to education is linked to better health outcomes and opportunities throughout life. Lifelong learning can keep the mind active and engaged.

Healthy Lifestyle Choices:

- Promote a healthy lifestyle with balanced nutrition, physical activity, and stress management from childhood onward. Avoiding tobacco, alcohol, and drugs is crucial.

Mental and Emotional Health

- Nurturing mental and emotional well-being is essential at every age. Teaching emotional intelligence and coping skills can have long-lasting benefits.

Regular Check-Ups and Preventive Care:

- Regular medical check-ups and preventive care help identify health issues early and allow for interventions to promote longevity.

Safety and Injury Prevention:

- Promote safety awareness to prevent accidents and injuries, which can have long-term consequences.

Healthy Relationships:

- Encourage the development of healthy, supportive relationships, as social connections contribute to emotional well-being and longevity.

Adulthood:

- Continuation of healthy habits from childhood and adolescence is vital. Manage stress and work-life balance, and maintain a focus on physical fitness.

Chronic Disease Prevention:

- Address risk factors for chronic diseases through regular screenings and lifestyle choices.

Healthy Diet:

- Adopt a balanced diet that meets nutritional needs. Avoid overconsumption and practice portion control.

Mental Fitness:

- Maintain cognitive health through lifelong learning, brain exercises, and social engagement.

Financial Planning:

- Plan for financial security to reduce stress and ensure a comfortable retirement.

Active Aging:

- Continue to be physically active in later life to maintain strength, balance, and overall health.

Community Engagement:

- Participate in community activities and support systems to foster a sense of belonging and purpose.

Mental and Emotional Health Support:

•Access mental health services and emotional support as needed. Addressing mental health concerns can improve overall well-being.

Preventive Health Measures:

- Stay up-to-date with vaccinations and health screenings.

Healthy Habits in Old Age:

- Continue to prioritize a balanced diet, physical activity, and regular medical check-ups in old age.

Quality of Life in Retirement:

- Plan for a fulfilling retirement, including hobbies, volunteer work, and staying socially connected.

End-of-Life Planning:

- Discuss and document end-of-life preferences, including medical care and funeral arrangements.

Longevity across the lifespan involves taking a proactive approach to health, well-being, and life satisfaction at every stage of life. By addressing various aspects of health and life fulfillment, individuals can increase their chances of living a long, healthy, and fulfilling life. It's important to seek guidance from healthcare professionals and experts in aging to make informed choices and maintain a high quality of life throughout the years.

Longevity for Children and Adolescents

Promoting longevity for children and adolescents involves instilling healthy habits and providing a supportive environment to set the foundation for a long and healthy life. Here are some key considerations for fostering longevity in younger individuals:

Healthy Nutrition: Encourage a balanced diet that includes a variety of fruits, vegetables, whole grains, lean proteins, and dairy products. Limit sugary and processed foods.

Physical Activity: Promote regular physical activity to help maintain a healthy weight, build strong bones and muscles, and improve cardiovascular health.

Limit Screen Time: Set reasonable limits on screen time, including television, computer, and mobile device usage. Excessive screen time is linked to a sedentary lifestyle.

Adequate Sleep: Ensure children and adolescents get the recommended amount of sleep for their age. Quality sleep is crucial for physical and mental development.

Regular Check-Ups: Schedule regular medical check-ups and vaccinations to monitor overall health and prevent illnesses.

Immunizations: Keep up to date with immunizations to protect against common childhood diseases.

Emotional Well-Being: Promote emotional health by encouraging open communication, teaching coping skills, and addressing stress and anxiety.

Tobacco and Substance Use Prevention: Educate children and adolescents about the risks of tobacco, alcohol, and drug use. Create a supportive, non-judgmental environment for discussions.

Safety Awareness: Teach safety precautions, such as the importance of wearing seatbelts, helmets, and other safety gear.

School and Education: Support education and learning. A good education is linked to better health outcomes and opportunities in adulthood.

Healthy Relationships: Teach children about the importance of healthy, respectful relationships and the consequences of bullying or abusive behavior.

Community Engagement: Encourage community involvement and volunteering to foster a sense of belonging and social responsibility.

Life Skills: Teach practical life skills, such as cooking, time management, and money management, which are important for self-sufficiency.

Body Image and Self-Esteem: Promote a positive body image and self-esteem by emphasizing the importance of self-acceptance and individuality.

Preventive Healthcare Education: Educate children and adolescents about the value of preventive healthcare measures, such as vaccinations and screenings.

Balanced Schedules: Help children and adolescents balance their schedules to avoid excessive stress and overcommitment.

Limit Exposure to Environmental Toxins: Minimize exposure to environmental toxins and pollutants by ensuring clean air and water at home and in the community.

Positive Role Models: Be a positive role model for healthy habits and behaviors. Children often learn by example.

Promoting longevity in children and adolescents is about equipping them with the knowledge, skills, and habits needed to lead a long, healthy, and fulfilling life. The early establishment of healthy routines and the nurturing of physical, mental, and emotional well-being lay the foundation for a lifetime of well-being. Parents, caregivers, and educators play a crucial role in imparting these values and practices.

Adult Health and Longevity

Adult health and longevity depend on maintaining a healthy lifestyle and addressing specific health considerations that arise during the adult years. Here are key factors to consider for promoting adult health and longevity:

Healthy Eating: Continue to maintain a balanced diet rich in fruits, vegetables, whole grains, lean proteins, and healthy fats. Pay attention to portion control to manage calorie intake.

Regular Physical Activity: Engage in regular physical activity to maintain a healthy weight, strengthen muscles and bones, and reduce the risk of chronic diseases.

Stress Management: Develop effective stress management techniques, such as meditation, mindfulness, yoga, or deep breathing exercises. Chronic stress can negatively impact health.

Tobacco and Alcohol Avoidance: Avoid or limit tobacco and alcohol consumption to reduce the risk of cancer, cardiovascular diseases, and other health problems.

Mental Health Care: Prioritize mental and emotional well-being. Seek professional help if needed and practice self-care for mental health.

Regular Check-Ups: Continue to schedule regular medical check-ups to monitor health and detect any issues early.

Preventive Health Measures: Stay up-to-date with vaccinations, screenings, and preventive health measures recommended for your age group.

Chronic Disease Prevention: Address risk factors for chronic diseases through lifestyle choices and regular health screenings.

Heart Health: Manage cardiovascular health through a heart-healthy diet, regular exercise, and routine blood pressure and cholesterol checks.

Diabetes Management: If you have diabetes or are at risk, carefully manage your blood sugar through medication, diet, and exercise.

Bone Health: Pay attention to bone health by ensuring an adequate intake of calcium and vitamin D, and engage in weight-bearing exercises to reduce the risk of osteoporosis.

Sexual Health: Maintain sexual health through regular check-ups, safe practices, and open communication with partners and healthcare providers.

Screenings for Age-Related Conditions: Adhere to recommended screenings for age-related conditions, such as mammograms for breast cancer and colonoscopies for colorectal cancer.

Weight Management: Manage weight to prevent obesity, which is a risk factor for various chronic diseases.

Life Purpose and Fulfillment: Continue to pursue a sense of purpose and fulfillment in adulthood, which can enhance mental and emotional well-being.

Social Connections: Foster and maintain strong social connections and relationships, which contribute to emotional well-being.

Career and Work-Life Balance: Strive for a balance between career and personal life to reduce stress and maintain overall well-being.

Preventive Measures for Environmental Health: Be aware of environmental toxins and pollutants that may affect health and take steps to minimize exposure.

Financial Planning: Plan for financial security, especially as you approach retirement, to reduce financial stress and ensure a comfortable lifestyle.

Active Aging: Stay physically and mentally active in later years to promote overall health and maintain independence.

Adult health and longevity are the result of consistent healthy habits and regular monitoring of health indicators. Prioritizing health and well-being at each stage of adulthood can lead to a longer and more fulfilling life.

Healthy Aging for Seniors

Healthy aging for seniors involves strategies and practices that promote physical, mental, and emotional well-being in later life. These are key considerations for seniors to achieve and maintain healthy aging:

Consume a balanced diet that includes plenty of fruits, vegetables, whole grains, lean proteins, and healthy fats. Adequate nutrition is essential for maintaining energy and overall health. Stay well-hydrated by drinking sufficient water throughout the day. Dehydration can lead to various health issues.

Engage in regular physical activity, including activities that improve strength, balance, and flexibility. This can help prevent falls and maintain mobility. Continue to schedule regular medical check-ups and screenings to monitor health and detect age-related conditions early.

If you take medications, follow your healthcare provider's instructions and adhere to your medication regimen. If you have chronic health conditions, actively manage them through lifestyle choices, medication, and regular follow-ups.

Maintain cardiovascular health by managing blood pressure, cholesterol levels, and adopting a heart-healthy diet. Pay attention to bone health by ensuring an adequate intake of calcium and vitamin D, and continue weight-bearing exercises to prevent osteoporosis.

Prioritize mental and emotional well-being by engaging in activities that keep the mind active, seeking emotional support when needed, and practicing stress management techniques. Promote quality sleep through good sleep hygiene practices. Address sleep issues with your healthcare provider.

Maintain social connections and stay engaged with friends, family, and your community. Strong social ties are associated with better emotional health. Seek a sense of purpose and fulfillment in retirement years through hobbies, volunteer work, or pursuing personal interests.

Stay up-to-date with vaccinations and screenings appropriate for your age and health status. Ensure a safe home environment by removing tripping hazards, installing handrails, and using assistive devices as needed.

Schedule regular eye and hearing exams to address vision and hearing changes. Maintain good oral hygiene and visit the dentist regularly, as oral health can impact overall health.

Take steps to prevent falls, such as using proper footwear, keeping a clutter-free home, and participating in balance exercises. Plan for financial security in retirement to reduce financial stress and ensure a comfortable lifestyle.

Discuss and document end-of-life preferences, including medical care and funeral arrangements. Engage in lifelong learning by attending classes, reading, or participating in educational activities to keep the mind sharp.

Healthy aging for seniors involves maintaining a high quality of life, staying active, and promoting well-being. These strategies can contribute to a fulfilling and rewarding later life.

End-of-Life Planning

End-of-life planning is a process that involves making decisions about your preferences for medical care, financial matters, and personal affairs as you approach the end of your life. This planning ensures that your wishes are respected and that your loved ones are informed and supported. Here are key components of end-of-life planning:

Advance Directives: Create advance directives, which include a living will and a healthcare proxy. A living will outline your medical treatment preferences, while a healthcare proxy designates someone to make medical decisions for you if you're unable to do so.

Do Not Resuscitate (DNR) Order: Discuss and establish a Do Not Resuscitate (DNR) order if you have specific preferences regarding CPR in case of cardiac arrest.

Power of Attorney: Designate a durable power of attorney for financial matters. This person can make financial decisions on your behalf if you become incapacitated.

Will and Estate Planning: Draft a will to specify how your assets and possessions should be distributed after your death. Consider estate planning to minimize tax implications and provide for your beneficiaries.

Funeral and Burial Preferences: Outline your preferences for funeral arrangements, including burial or cremation, memorial services, and other related matters.

Organ Donation: If you wish to donate organs or tissues after your death, make your intentions known and consider registering as an organ donor.

Digital Assets: Include digital assets in your planning, such as passwords and access to online accounts or social media profiles. Determine how these should be managed or closed after your passing.

Guardianship for Dependents: If you have dependents, establish guardianship arrangements to ensure their care and well-being in case you're no longer able to provide for them.

Family Discussions: Have open and honest discussions with family members or close friends about your end-of-life preferences. Ensure they are aware of your wishes and where to find important documents.

Advance Care Planning: Discuss your values and preferences for end-of-life care with healthcare providers and family members. This can help guide medical decisions if you become unable to communicate your wishes.

Insurance and Financial Review: Review your life insurance policies, retirement accounts, and financial assets to ensure your beneficiaries are up-to-date and your wishes are clear.

Legal Assistance: Consult with an attorney experienced in estate planning and end-of-life matters to ensure your documents are legally sound and reflect your intentions.

End-of-life planning can provide peace of mind for both you and your loved ones. It ensures that your final wishes are honored, eases the decision-making burden on family members, and reduces the likelihood of disputes. The planning process can be emotionally challenging, but it is an important aspect of responsible financial and personal management.

Legacy and Life Reflection

Legacy and life reflection are meaningful aspects of end-of-life planning and a way to leave a lasting impact on the world and those you care about. They involve reflecting on your life, values, and the legacy you wish to leave behind. Below are key considerations for legacy and life reflection:

Reflect on Your Values:
- Take time to think about your core values, beliefs, and the principles that have guided your life.

Life Story and Memories:
- Share your life story and memories with loved ones. Consider writing a memoir, creating an oral history, or recording your experiences.

Personal Philosophy:

- Reflect on your personal philosophy, including your thoughts on life, death, happiness, and fulfillment.

Family History:

- Document and share your family's history and traditions to ensure they are passed down through generations.

Life Lessons:

- Share the wisdom and life lessons you've gained from your experiences. Consider creating a document or series of letters to convey these insights.

Letters to Loved Ones:

- Write heartfelt letters to your family and friends, expressing your love, gratitude, and advice for their future.

Philanthropy and Charitable Giving:

- Consider how you can contribute to causes and organizations that align with your values. Share your philanthropic goals with family members and leave a legacy of giving.

Artistic or Creative Expression:

- Express your thoughts and feelings through artistic endeavors, such as writing, painting, music, or any form of creative expression.

Family Heirlooms and Treasures:

- Identify and document family heirlooms, their significance, and to whom you would like to pass them down.

Ethical Will:
- Create an ethical will, a document that conveys your moral and ethical values to your heirs and loved ones.

Legacy Projects:
- Consider initiating or participating in legacy projects that reflect your passions or interests, such as community service, education, or artistic endeavors.

Photo Albums and Family Records:
- Organize family photos and records, ensuring they are accessible to future generations.

Digital Legacy:
- Make arrangements for your digital legacy, including the management and preservation of digital assets, such as photos, documents, and online accounts.

Environmental Legacy:
- Reflect on your relationship with the environment and consider actions that support sustainability and ecological responsibility.

Education and Values Transmission:
- Share educational materials and resources that reflect your values and beliefs with younger generations.

Letters of Forgiveness and Reconciliation:

- Consider writing letters of forgiveness and reconciliation to resolve any past conflicts or misunderstandings.

Reflection and Personal Growth:
- Embrace this phase of life for personal growth, introspection, and contemplation of your unique journey.

Legacy and life reflection provide an opportunity to pass on your values, experiences, and wisdom to future generations. It allows you to create a lasting impact and ensure that your legacy endures in the hearts and minds of those who matter most to you. Engaging in these activities can be a profoundly meaningful and therapeutic process as you approach the later stages of life.

Chapter 8

Longevity Hacks in a Changing World

Longevity in a changing world presents both opportunities and challenges. As society and technology evolve, individuals have the potential to lead longer, healthier lives, but they also face new complexities and considerations. These are key factors to consider when thinking about longevity in a changing world:

Medical breakthroughs and innovations continue to extend life expectancies and improve the quality of life for older individuals. Access to cutting-edge healthcare is becoming more widespread. Greater awareness of preventive healthcare and wellness practices can help individuals proactively manage their health and reduce the risk of chronic diseases.

Technology plays a vital role in extending longevity through telehealth, wearable health devices, and digital health records that enable better monitoring and management of health. Emphasis is shifting from simply living longer to maintaining a high quality of life in older age. This includes physical and cognitive well-being, emotional health, and social connections.

As people live longer, they are redefining retirement and seeking opportunities for lifelong learning and part-time work to stay engaged and fulfilled. Longevity necessitates careful financial planning and saving for retirement to ensure financial security in later years.

The recognition of the importance of mental and emotional health is growing, with greater emphasis on reducing stigma and seeking help when needed. Strong social connections and support systems are vital for well-being in later life. Efforts to combat social isolation are on the rise.

Addressing environmental sustainability is crucial for the well-being of current and future generations. Protecting the environment ensures a healthier world for older individuals. Aging in place, or living independently at home, is becoming more attainable with the assistance of technology and support services.

Diverse cultural backgrounds and generational perspectives play a role in how individuals approach aging and longevity. Discussions about end-of-life preferences and choices, including palliative care and euthanasia, are becoming more common.

Ethical dilemmas and legal considerations, such as healthcare decision-making and elder abuse, require attention and resolution.
Managing and preserving digital legacies, including online profiles and social media accounts, is an emerging aspect of end-of-life planning.

Active participation in the community and civic engagement can provide a sense of purpose and connection for older individuals.
The aging population is a global phenomenon, with implications for healthcare systems, pensions, and intergenerational relationships.

Longevity in a changing world is a multifaceted concept that requires adaptability and informed decision-making. It is essential to stay informed, make conscious choices about lifestyle and healthcare, and engage in discussions about end-of-life preferences and environmental sustainability. Embracing these changes and opportunities can lead to a longer, more fulfilling life in an evolving world.

Environmental Sustainability

Environmental sustainability refers to the responsible use of Earth's natural resources and the protection of the environment to ensure its health and well-being for current and future generations. It involves practices that help maintain ecological balance, minimize waste, and reduce negative impacts on the environment. Key components of environmental sustainability include:

Minimize the use of non-renewable resources, such as fossil fuels and minerals, and promote the responsible use of renewable resources, including forests, water, and soil. Reduce energy consumption by using energy-efficient technologies and practices, such as LED lighting, improved insulation, and sustainable transportation. Invest in and promote the use of renewable energy sources, such as solar, wind, and hydroelectric power, to reduce greenhouse gas emissions and dependence on fossil fuels.

Minimize waste generation and promote recycling and composting to reduce the amount of waste sent to landfills. Protect and preserve ecosystems and wildlife habitats to maintain biodiversity and prevent the extinction of species.

Promote environmentally friendly agricultural practices that minimize soil erosion, reduce chemical pesticide use, and support healthy soil and crop diversity. Maintain and improve water quality by reducing pollution and protecting water sources. Promote clean air through reduced emissions and better air quality management.

Encourage public transportation, carpooling, biking, and walking to reduce traffic congestion and emissions from fossil fuel-powered vehicles. Design cities and communities that are walkable, bike-friendly, and energy-efficient, reducing the need for long commutes and excessive energy consumption.

Practice the "3 Rs" to reduce waste: reduce consumption, reuse items when possible, and recycle materials like paper, glass, and plastic. Promote environmental education and awareness to encourage individuals and communities to make sustainable choices.

Advocate for and support policies and regulations that protect the environment, including emissions standards, conservation laws, and sustainable land use planning. Invest in and support the development of green technologies, such as electric vehicles, renewable energy systems, and energy-efficient appliances.

Make conscious consumer choices by buying products with minimal environmental impact, supporting eco-friendly brands, and reducing single-use plastics. Protect wilderness areas and natural landscapes from development and industrial activities to preserve their ecological value.

Implement eco-friendly practices in everyday life, such as reducing water consumption, composting organic waste, and using eco-friendly cleaning products. Address climate change by reducing greenhouse gas emissions and supporting initiatives to limit global temperature rise.

Environmental sustainability is vital for the health and well-being of the planet and its inhabitants. It requires a collective effort, from individuals and communities to governments and businesses, to protect and preserve natural resources and maintain a balanced and thriving environment for future generations.

Technological Advancements

Technological advancements refer to the continual progress and development of technologies that have the potential to improve various aspects of human life, from healthcare and communication to transportation and industry. Here are some key areas of technological advancements:

Information Technology: Advancements in computing power, software, and networking have led to faster data processing, improved cybersecurity, and the expansion of cloud computing.

Artificial Intelligence (AI): AI and machine learning have made significant strides, enabling applications in natural language processing, autonomous vehicles, healthcare diagnostics, and more.

Biotechnology: Biotechnological innovations have given rise to breakthroughs in gene editing, personalized medicine, and advancements in pharmaceuticals.

Robotics: Robotics technologies are used in manufacturing, healthcare, and even personal assistance, with applications ranging from surgical robots to home automation.

Renewable Energy: Progress in renewable energy sources, such as solar and wind power, is contributing to sustainable energy production and reducing reliance on fossil fuels.

Electric Vehicles (EVs): Electric vehicle technology is improving, with longer battery life, faster charging, and broader adoption, contributing to reduced emissions in the transportation sector.

Space Exploration: Technological advancements in space exploration are enabling missions to Mars, lunar exploration, and the study of exoplanets.

Healthcare Technology: Telemedicine, wearable health devices, and electronic health records are transforming healthcare delivery and patient management.

Biometrics: Biometric technologies, including fingerprint recognition, facial recognition, and iris scanning, are being used for security and identity verification.

Blockchain Technology: Blockchain is revolutionizing industries such as finance, supply chain, and healthcare with secure and transparent record-keeping.

Quantum Computing: Quantum computing has the potential to solve complex problems faster than classical computers, with applications in cryptography, materials science, and more.

Smart Cities: Smart city technologies are enhancing urban living with IoT-connected infrastructure, improved transportation systems, and energy efficiency.

Augmented and Virtual Reality (AR/VR): AR and VR technologies are changing how we experience entertainment, education, and even remote work.

3D Printing: 3D printing is being used for rapid prototyping, custom manufacturing, and medical applications, including prosthetics and dental devices.

Cybersecurity: Advancements in cybersecurity are crucial to protect digital assets and sensitive information from cyber threats.

Environmental Technologies: Technologies for waste reduction, water purification, and air quality improvement are contributing to a more sustainable future.

Agricultural Technology: Agtech innovations are improving crop yield, livestock management, and food supply chain efficiency.

Transportation Technologies: Autonomous vehicles and high-speed transportation systems like hyperloop are changing the way people and goods move.

These technological advancements are continually reshaping industries, economies, and everyday life. They offer opportunities for improving efficiency, solving complex problems, and addressing global challenges, but they also raise ethical and regulatory considerations that need to be addressed to ensure responsible and beneficial use.

Global Health Challenges

Global health challenges are complex and multifaceted issues that affect the well-being and healthcare of people worldwide. These challenges often transcend national borders and require collaborative efforts among governments, organizations, and communities to address. Some of the major global health challenges include:

Infectious Diseases

- Infectious diseases like HIV/AIDS, malaria, tuberculosis, and emerging infectious diseases (e.g., Ebola, Zika, COVID-19) continue to pose significant global health threats.

Vaccine Hesitancy

- Vaccine hesitancy and resistance to immunization efforts can lead to outbreaks of vaccine-preventable diseases.

Antibiotic Resistance

- The rise of antibiotic-resistant bacteria threatens our ability to treat common infections, making healthcare less effective and more expensive.

Non-Communicable Diseases (NCDs)

- NCDs such as heart disease, cancer, diabetes, and respiratory diseases are responsible for the majority of global deaths, with lifestyle factors contributing to their rise.

Mental Health

- Mental health disorders, including depression, anxiety, and stress-related conditions, are a significant global health concern with widespread implications for well-being.

Maternal and Child Health

- High maternal and child mortality rates persist in many parts of the world due to factors like inadequate healthcare access, malnutrition, and infectious diseases.

Access to Healthcare

- Access to quality healthcare services remains a challenge, particularly in low- and middle-income countries where resources are limited.

Healthcare Disparities

- Disparities in health outcomes exist along socioeconomic, racial, and regional lines, leading to unequal access to care and health outcomes.

Climate Change and Health

- Climate change contributes to extreme weather events, the spread of vector-borne diseases, and the displacement of communities, impacting public health.

Food Security and Nutrition

- Insufficient access to nutritious food and poor nutrition lead to malnutrition and related health issues.

Water and Sanitation

- Lack of access to clean water and proper sanitation facilities contributes to waterborne diseases and poor health.

Global Health Security

- Outbreaks of infectious diseases, as seen with COVID-19, highlight the need for global health security measures and rapid response systems.

Substance Abuse and Addiction
- Substance abuse, including alcohol and drug addiction, is a global health concern with serious social and health consequences.

Aging Populations
- Many countries are experiencing aging populations, which present unique healthcare challenges, including long-term care and chronic disease management.

Conflict and Displacement
- Armed conflicts and humanitarian crises disrupt healthcare systems, displace populations, and create conditions for the spread of disease.

Global Healthcare Workforce
- Shortages of healthcare workers, particularly in underserved areas, limit access to care and healthcare system capacity.

Addressing these global health challenges requires a comprehensive and collaborative approach involving governments, international organizations, non-governmental organizations (NGOs), healthcare professionals, and communities. Priorities include building robust healthcare infrastructure, improving health education and awareness, advancing research and development, and promoting policies that prioritize health equity and social determinants of health. Efforts to address these challenges contribute to a healthier and more equitable world for all.

Longevity and Social Equity

Longevity and social equity are closely intertwined, as access to resources, opportunities, and quality healthcare significantly impact an individual's lifespan and overall well-being. Here's how longevity and social equity are connected:

Health Disparities

- Socially disadvantaged groups often experience health disparities, including higher rates of chronic diseases, limited access to healthcare, and reduced life expectancy. Improving social equity is critical to addressing these disparities and extending longevity.

Access to Healthcare

- Social equity plays a vital role in ensuring equal access to healthcare services. Disparities in healthcare access, affordability, and quality can directly affect an individual's ability to receive timely and appropriate medical care, which in turn influences their longevity.

Social Determinants of Health

- Social factors such as income, education, employment, housing, and access to healthy food and clean water are known as social determinants of health. These factors greatly impact a person's health and longevity. Addressing social determinants of health is essential for achieving social equity.

Environmental Justice

- Vulnerable communities often face greater exposure to environmental hazards, such as pollution and climate change, which can have adverse effects on health and longevity. Achieving social equity involves addressing environmental justice concerns to protect the well-being of all individuals.

Education and Literacy

- Access to education and health literacy are key components of social equity. Individuals with higher levels of education and health literacy tend to make more informed health decisions, leading to better health outcomes and longer lives.

Income and Economic Security

- People with lower incomes may experience financial stress, reduced access to healthcare, and increased vulnerability to adverse health conditions. Efforts to reduce income inequality and provide economic security can positively impact longevity.

Nutrition and Food Security

- Food security and access to nutritious, affordable food are essential for maintaining good health and longevity. Initiatives to address food deserts and improve nutritional equity are critical for social well-being.

Aging and Elder Care

- Older individuals often face unique challenges related to social equity, including access to quality elder care, social services, and financial security during retirement. Ensuring that aging populations receive support is vital for promoting longevity.

Cultural Competence

- Achieving social equity in healthcare includes recognizing and addressing cultural and language barriers that can affect the delivery of care. Culturally competent healthcare ensures that individuals from diverse backgrounds receive appropriate services and support.

Mental Health Equity

- Social equity extends to mental health, encompassing access to mental health services, reducing stigma, and addressing the unique mental health challenges faced by different communities.

Community and Social Support

- Strong social networks and community support systems are essential for well-being and longevity. Building and maintaining these networks can be influenced by social equity factors.

Preventive Healthcare and Screening

- Socially equitable access to preventive healthcare services, including vaccinations, screenings, and wellness check-ups, can help detect and address health issues before they become severe.

Promoting social equity and longevity involves addressing systemic inequities in healthcare, education, employment, housing, and more. It calls for policies and interventions that reduce disparities, promote equal opportunities, and ensure that everyone, regardless of their background, has the chance to live a long, healthy, and fulfilling life. Achieving social equity in longevity is not only a matter of fairness but also essential for creating a healthier and more sustainable society.

A Future of Longevity

The future of longevity holds exciting possibilities and challenges as people around the world continue to live longer, healthier lives. These are some key aspects of what the future of longevity may look like:

Extended Life Expectancy: Advances in healthcare, preventive medicine, and lifestyle changes are likely to continue extending human life expectancy. Living well into the 80s, 90s, and even over 100 could become more common.

Healthy Aging: The emphasis will shift from merely extending life to enhancing the quality of life in old age. Efforts will focus on promoting physical, mental, and emotional well-being.

Personalized Medicine: Advances in genomics and biotechnology will enable personalized medical treatments tailored to an individual's genetic makeup, lifestyle, and health history.

Anti-Aging Therapies: Research into anti-aging therapies, such as senolytics and regenerative medicine, may slow down the aging process and reduce age-related diseases.

Digital Health: Technology will play a significant role in healthcare, with telemedicine, wearable health devices, and AI-driven diagnostics becoming more prevalent.

Elder-Friendly Cities: Urban planning will cater to the needs of aging populations, creating age-friendly cities with accessible infrastructure, healthcare, and social services.

Nutrition and Lifestyle: There will be a greater focus on nutrition, exercise, and lifestyle as means to maintain health and vitality in older age.

Cognitive Health: Cognitive health and brain fitness will be important, with innovations in brain training and therapies for neurodegenerative diseases.

Biological Rejuvenation: Research into biological rejuvenation and extending "health spans" may revolutionize aging and health.

Regulatory Challenges: As anti-aging and longevity treatments develop, regulatory bodies will need to adapt to ensure safety and efficacy.

Healthcare Access: Addressing health care access disparities and ensuring that advancements benefit all socio-economic groups is crucial.

Environmental Sustainability: Promoting a sustainable environment is essential, as the environmental impact of a growing elderly population must be managed responsibly.

Social Connections: Encouraging strong social connections and addressing social isolation in aging populations is vital for well-being.

Ethical Considerations: Discussions on ethical dilemmas, end-of-life choices, and the use of emerging technologies in longevity will be important.

Mental Health Support: Greater awareness and support for mental health, particularly in older adults, will be essential for promoting overall well-being.

Global Perspective: Longevity is a global issue, and challenges and solutions will vary across cultures and regions.

The future of longevity is exciting, but it also raises important ethical, social, and healthcare questions. As societies adapt to an aging population, it will be essential to create policies and systems that promote health and well-being across all age groups and ensure that the benefits of extended life are accessible to everyone. Ultimately, the future of longevity has the potential to transform not only our individual lives but also society as a whole.

Summary

The Journey to a Longer, Healthier Life

Finally, the journey to a longer, healthier life is a path filled with choices, challenges, and opportunities. Throughout this book, we've explored "How not to get aged," delving into a wide range of topics aimed at helping you achieve a fulfilling and vital existence. Below are takeaways to sum up "How not to get aged" journey:

- Balanced Diet: A nutritious, well-rounded diet is the cornerstone of good health and longevity.

- Portion Control and Mindful Eating: Be conscious of what and how much you eat, focusing on quality over quantity.

- Superfoods for Longevity: Incorporate nutrient-dense superfoods into your meals for added health benefits.

- Hydration: Proper hydration is essential for bodily functions and overall health.

- Role of Supplements: Supplements can complement your diet, but they should be used thoughtfully and in consultation with a healthcare provider.

- Regular Exercise: Physical activity is key to longevity, so find enjoyable ways to keep moving.

- Cardiovascular Health: Maintain a strong heart through exercise, a heart-healthy diet, and stress management.

- Strength Training: Building muscle strength and bone density is essential for healthy aging.

- Flexibility and Mobility: Stay limber to prevent injury and maintain functional independence.

- Mind-Body Connection: Your mental and emotional health are inseparable from your physical well-being.

- Mental and Emotional Well-Being: Prioritize mental health, seek support when needed, and manage stress effectively.

- Social Connections: A strong social network is a vital aspect of longevity and well-being.

- The Power of Positive Thinking: A positive outlook can improve your health and help you overcome challenges.

- The Science of Sleep: Quality sleep is essential for mental and physical health.

Sleep and Rest: Prioritize restful sleep and create a sleep-friendly environment.

Napping for Longevity: Strategic napping can boost alertness and overall well-being.

Managing Insomnia: Address sleep disturbances for better quality rest.

Lifestyle and Habits: Make conscious choices to support your health and well-being.

Quitting Smoking: Smoking cessation is one of the most significant steps toward better health.

Reducing Alcohol Consumption: Moderation in alcohol consumption is key to health and longevity.

Avoiding Harmful Chemicals: Minimize exposure to harmful chemicals and pollutants.

Living a Purposeful Life: Find meaning and purpose in your daily activities.

Preventive Healthcare: Regular check-ups and screenings can detect and address health issues early.

Legacy and Life Reflection: Share your wisdom, values, and life experiences to leave a meaningful legacy.

End-of-Life Planning: Plan for your future and communicate your preferences with loved ones.

Environmental Sustainability: Protect the environment for the benefit of current and future generations.

Technological Advancements: Embrace and utilize technology for improved healthcare and quality of life.

Global Health Challenges: Be aware of global health issues and contribute to solutions.

Longevity and Social Equity: Advocate for equal access to healthcare and well-being for all.

A Future of Longevity: Look forward to a future where extended, high-quality life is achievable.

Your journey to a longer, healthier life is an ongoing process. It's about making informed choices, nurturing your physical and mental health, and embracing the opportunities and challenges of the future. Note that the choices you make today can influence the quality and duration of your life.

Appendix

Key Terms and Definitions

1. Balanced Diet: A diet that provides essential nutrients in the right proportions to support overall health and well-being.

2. Superfoods: Nutrient-rich foods that offer exceptional health benefits due to their high content of vitamins, minerals, and antioxidants.

3. Portion Control: Managing the amount of food you eat in a single sitting to avoid overeating and maintain a healthy weight.

4. Mindful Eating: Paying close attention to the experience of eating, including the taste, texture, and sensations, to savor and enjoy food while also recognizing hunger and fullness cues.

5. Supplements: Products such as vitamins, minerals, and herbal extracts taken as a supplement to the diet to address nutritional deficiencies or promote health.

6. Cardiovascular Health: The health of the heart and blood vessels, essential for proper circulation and overall well-being.

7. Strength Training: A form of exercise that involves resistance or weight training to build muscle strength and endurance.

8. Flexibility and Mobility: The ability to move joints and muscles through their full range of motion, promoting physical health and preventing injury.

9. Mind-Body Connection: The interrelationship between mental and emotional well-being and physical health.

10. Mental and Emotional Well-Being: The state of emotional and psychological health, encompassing mental health, stress management, and emotional balance.

11. Stress Management: Strategies and techniques to cope with and reduce stress, promoting mental and physical health.

12. Social Connections: The relationships and social networks that provide support, companionship, and a sense of belonging.

13. Positive Thinking: An optimistic mindset that emphasizes constructive and hopeful thoughts, which can contribute to better health and well-being.

14. Sleep Hygiene: Practices and habits that promote good sleep quality, including creating a sleep-friendly environment and adhering to a regular sleep schedule.

15. Napping: A short period of sleep during the day, which can offer rest and mental rejuvenation.

16. Lifestyle and Habits: The daily choices and routines that impact overall health, well-being, and longevity.

17. Preventive Healthcare: Medical practices and interventions aimed at preventing illness or detecting health issues at an early, treatable stage.

18. Social Equity: The concept of fairness and justice in the distribution of resources and opportunities across different societal groups.

19. Environmental Sustainability: The responsible use of Earth's resources and the protection of the environment to ensure long-term well-being.

20. Technological Advancements: The continual progress in technology and innovation that leads to new tools, devices, and systems for improving various aspects of human life.

21. Global Health Challenges: Complex and widespread health issues that affect populations across the world, often requiring international cooperation to address.

22. Longevity: The state or quality of living a long and healthy life, often associated with a high life expectancy.

These definitions provide a foundation for understanding the concepts and practices discussed in the book. They are essential for making informed decisions and taking proactive steps toward a longer, healthier life.

www.ingramcontent.com/pod-product-compliance
Lightning Source LLC
Chambersburg PA
CBHW070757260726
48660CB00005B/1657